THE FUNCTIONAL APPROACH TO HYPOTHYROIDISM

THE FUNCTIONAL APPROACH TO HYPOTHYROIDISM

Bridging Traditional & Alternative Treatment Approaches for **Total Patient Wellness**

KENNETH R. BLANCHARD, PH.D., M.D.

hatherleigh

The Functional Approach to Hypothyroidism

Hatherleigh Press is committed to preserving and protecting the natural resources of the earth. Environmentally responsible and sustainable practices are embraced within the company's mission statement. Hatherleigh Press is a member of the Publishers Earth Alliance, committed to preserving and protecting the natural resources of the planet while developing a sustainable business model for the book publishing industry.

DISCLAIMER
This book does not give legal or medical advice. Always consult your doctor, lawyer, and other professionals. The ideas and suggestions contained in this book are not intended as a substitute for consulting with a physician. All matters regarding your health require medical supervision.

Library of Congress Cataloging-in-Publication Data is available.
ISBN: 978-1-57826-387-5

Cover Design by Dede Cummings Designs
Interior Design by Dede Cummings Designs

Printed in the United States

10 9 8 7 6 5 4 3 2

hatherleigh

www.hatherleighpress.com

The Only Thing That Matters Is . . .
Does It Work or Doesn't It Work?

All truth passes through three stages. First, it is ridiculed, then it is attacked and finally, it is regarded as self-evident.

—Schopenauer

ACKNOWLEDGEMENTS

THIS BOOK AND my career have been possible because of several loyal and dedicated employees over the years. Elisabeth Daniels, Carol Shander, and Kay Kearney got me through some difficult times in the early and middle portions of my career. In recent years, Maggie MacLeod, Cheryl Gaucher, and Barry Heller have served me well and protected me from the many stresses of running a medical practice. Many thanks to the staffs at Chatham Yacht Basin and (now) Pirate Cove Marina for making my excursions out on the ocean so pleasurable and restoring. Thanks to Tony Fiory, Jim Latimer, Bob Vernon, and my other MIT rowing colleagues, with whom I have shared the thrill of rowing 8-oared crew races again 45 years after the college experience. Many thanks also to Dennis Katz of Hopkinton Drug, whose compounding wizardry was extraordinarily helpful in this work. I have been extremely fortunate in having a wonderful family, which has spared me from some of the difficult experiences that many people face later in life. Many thanks also to Anna Krusinski and Christine Schultz of Hatherleigh Press for their expert editing suggestions. Lastly, I would like to thank the many loyal patients who have come to me from far and wide and have remained in my practice for many years, offering ultimate vindication to all the things I have done in this field.

CONTENTS

INTRODUCTION

THIS BOOK REPRESENTS the product of 33 years of medical practice, the first half of which was spent following the basic dogma about hypothyroidism that has been taught to all physicians since the 1970s. At the core of standard academic teaching in the field of hypothyroidism is the concept that the TSH (thyroid-stimulating hormone) test is the absolute "yes or no" test for the condition and its treatment, along with the belief that treatment with 100 percent T_4 is all that is needed because "T_4 is converted to T_3 in the body." As I started to question these teachings in my practice in the mid-1980s, I experienced a great deal of anxiety about going against the specific teachings of academic physicians whom I regard with great respect. What if a coincidental medical disaster were to happen to one of the patients in my practice while being treated the "wrong" way? I would have been the "local M.D." who was disobeying the rules of practice set down by eminent academic physicians with hundreds of publications on the subject. However, it has all worked out extremely well for me and my patients, and it is very clear to us that the standard teachings in the field are simply wrong or at best, incomplete. I would like to repeat a bit of philosophical wisdom from the introduction to my previous book: the only people who have absolute answers to anything in medicine are medical students, malpractice lawyers, and well-compensated expert witnesses. When desperate patients give this book to skeptical physicians, they will be met with cries of "anecdotal" and "no studies prove this." However, I will stand by all the assertions that I have made in this book and history will ultimately determine which side of the argument is right.

The contents of this book are informational. Treatment for a specific individual must be in the hands of their personal practitioner. Thyroid hormone replacement therapy is strictly by prescription, and for good reason.

CHAPTER 1

Why?

THIS BOOK is written for the millions of hypothyroid patients who have not been diagnosed or, if diagnosed, are treated poorly. Hypothyroidism is a disorder characterized by a wide array of symptoms but centered on fatigue caused by inadequate secretion of hormone by the thyroid gland located at the base of the neck. It is my assertion that the fundamental teachings in the field of hypothyroidism in the last 3 to 4 decades are largely wrong. Like-minded physicians and I have been dismissed by the academic leaders in this field because of the blind belief that anything that appears in a double-blind study in a major journal must be true, and anything that appears in a popular book like this one is dismissed as "anecdotal."

THE MYTHS OF HYPOTHYROIDISM

1. You can't be hypothyroid because your "TSH is within normal limits."
2. Nobody needs T_3 because T_4 gets converted to T_3 in the body.
3. Studies have proven that T_3 makes people worse rather than better.
4. Studies have proven that thyroid function has nothing to do with premenstrual syndrome (PMS).
5. If your TSH is normal, you cannot benefit from taking thyroid hormone.
6. There is no relation between fibromyalgia and hypothyroidism.
7. There is no benefit in seasonal adjustment of thyroid replacement therapy.
8. A "normal" TSH rules out hypothyroidism as a cause of infertility, miscarriage, or prematurity.
9. Postpartum depression has nothing to do with thyroid balance.
10. If you are "on thyroid" and your TSH is "normal," your symptoms cannot be related to hypothyroidism.
11. Hypothyroidism has nothing to do with susceptibility to motion sickness.

Ever since the 1970s the teaching has been that the TSH (thyroid-stimulating hormone) test is the absolute "gold standard" for assessing thyroid status. The normal range is usually given by laboratories as up to 4.5 to 5 or so and a patient is supposed to have a TSH higher than normal to make the proper diagnosis of hypothyroidism. Recently, the American Association of Clinical Endocrinologists has endorsed the idea that the upper limit of normal for TSH be set at 3.0. In my own practice since 1985, I have started over 1,000 patients on thyroid hormone without ever having an elevated TSH. The net result of this has been the tremendous success of my practice.. Another endocrinologist in my area recently published a thyroid book for lay people and, when asked by a magazine writer why he wrote the book, his reply was "there are popular books out there that are spreading misinformation about thyroid disease." While my book (*What Your Doctor May Not Tell You About Hypothyroidism*, Warner Books, 2004) was not specifically named by this author, I am sure he was referring to it as well as to others that have espoused the same ideas. His book no doubt gives the "party line" of the basic principles of the diagnosis and treatment of hypothyroidism that has been taught since the 1970s and that I believe are in desperate need of revision.

The two major thyroid hormones secreted by the thyroid gland are T_4 and T_3, and it has also been doctrine since the 1970s to state that "nobody needs T_3 because T_4 gets converted to T_3 in the body." Since 1990, I have routinely used T_3 in virtually all the patients in my practice and it has been extremely successful and without adverse effects. In particular, a number of studies published in the last few years have purported to "prove" that T_3 makes people worse rather than better. As will be discussed in detail later, I believe that these studies are classic "triple-blind" studies, that is, double-blind studies done by researchers who do not understand the subject they are researching. Although leading medical journals have published many studies that "prove" that the TSH is the absolute measure of thyroid function and that T_3 does not benefit patients, that does not make such assertions automatically true. Many studies in various fields have passed muster for publication in major journals only to be later proven wrong. For example, medical training in the 1970s taught that ulcer disease was caused by stomach acid due to stress, smoking, spices, and so on. In about 1980 a courageous Australian came along and asserted that ulcers were in fact caused by bacteria. He was roundly criticized for years, but his theory was eventually proven correct.

For the sake of our patients, I believe we need to junk the idea that laboratory numbers and journal articles tell you the absolute truth and that the results of empirical treatment on the basis of a physician's judgment are "anecdotal" and therefore not to be believed. Rather, we must move to what I would call a "functional" assessment of hypothyroidism. By this I mean that when a patient presents symptoms, all of which are compatible with hypothyroidism, if the physician then additionally finds some physical evidence suggesting hypothyroidism, this diagnosis should not be ruled out on the basis of a TSH test. Empirical trial of thyroid, although considered old-fashioned and disproven by typical academicians, actually represents the best way to go. If such a patient on empirical treatment feels unequivocally better after a few days or weeks on treatment, then that is in my opinion the closest that we can come to absolute answers in medicine. This approach has been extremely gratifying for hundreds of patients in my practice and anyone with an open mind who would like to sample the patients' opinions should do a Google search under my name.

What I have learned after 33 years in my practice, are some simple facts that should make the academic leaders in this field take notice (although they probably won't). At this time, I have never had a malpractice case in my entire career, I have approximately 250 patients in my practice who come to me from outside of New England, and I have 15 patients from foreign countries. I have about two hundred patients in my practice who came to me from the most eminent thyroid specialists in Boston (who have virtually none of my former patients). These are simple facts and I would like to hear the explanation of why these facts exist other than what I have been doing is working.

As my own career winds down, many of my patients are expressing anxiety about my retirement. It is time for the academicians to recognize openly that the large majority of their patients being treated with the standard 100 percent T_4 come into their offices complaining about how they feel.

Above all, I would like this book to be one that open-minded physicians and empowered patients can use as a manual toward better thyroid results. There is a great deal of benefit in tending to the many details of thyroid treatment. In this sense, I think that treating hypothyroidism resembles the relationship that physicians have with diabetes mellitus patients; that is, the patients take a great responsibility for day-to-day alterations in treatment. Ideally, patients with diabetes will take frequent blood sugar measurements and make minor insulin and food adjustments on their own. Treating hypothyroidism is not as complicated as treating diabetes mellitus, but I think that some of the same principles should apply. Patients can be on the type of T_4-T_3 mixtures that I recommend and still feel terrible, unless the dosage and T_4:T_3 ratios are optimal. Hence, one must be ready to try different dosages and different T_4:T_3 percentages until an optimum treatment point is reached. Since it is true that a significant minority of patients feel fine on 100 percent T_4 and a smaller number of patients feel well on thyroid extract (80:20 T_4:T_3), then it stands to reason that there will be people who are optimal at various points along the spectrum between 100:0 and 80:20 T_4:T_3.Thyroid extract is obtained from porcine thyroid glands and has been in use for over a century. In pill form, this is referred to as "Armour Thyroid." Thyroid extract is favored by some physicians because it is natural in origin, but the T_3 percentage is too high for this to be an effective long-term replacement therapy for most patients. Those patients and their physicians who take the message of this book seriously will wind up asking the fundamental question: *How can so many leaders in this field have been so wrong for so many years yet be absolutely adamant about their beliefs?*

No pretense is made for this book being a scholarly work with hundreds of references. Although many papers have been published with dozens or hundreds of references and so are labeled "scholarly" but they are fundamentally wrong. This approach is plainly taken to assist physicians who would like to review a few papers on the subject, but nowadays our empowered patients are often going directly to the journals themselves. The abbreviations used in this book are as follows:

JCEM, Journal of Clinical Endocrinology and Metabolism
NEJM, New England Journal of Medicine
BMJ, British Medicine Journal
AIM Annals of Internal Medicine

Throughout the book, I offer theories about the observations that we physicians make concerning our patients. As a scientist, I would like to believe that I can understand the basic reasons why certain things happen, but as a practitioner, all I really care about is what works. In other words, even if some theory I propose in this book is later proven to be wrong, I believe the only thing that really matters is whether or not a treatment variation based on that theory gives a better result. Many thyroid practitioners are likely to first learn about this book when it is handed to them by the desperate patients who are living with this condition. I would plead with those physicians to not casually discard the book; please look over the text, especially Chapter 2, and see if any of my concepts ring true for you. If you approach this book with an open mind, I believe you will come to understand that I know what I am talking about and that major changes in this field are long overdue.

CHAPTER 2

Observations

IN RECENT years, in my career as an endocrinologist I have received skeptical comments from colleagues, such as "he is overenthusiastic about thyroid," "no studies prove what he says," and so on. For those physicians who are open-minded enough to be reading this, I would like now to point out a number of observations that every physician who does this work makes virtually daily in his or her practice. If you are a patient reading this book and then passing it on to your physician, ask him or her to start with this chapter.

TIMING OF THYROID DOSES AND WEIGHT GAIN

We were all taught to "take thyroid hormones on an empty stomach first thing in the morning and wait one hour before taking any other pills or food." A simple fact clear to any physician is that the majority of patients started on thyroid actually gain weight rather than lose, as is the popular perception. These patients often report food cravings. It occurred to me that these cravings may be related to T_4 coming into direct contact with the walls of the stomach. I had such patients take their T_4 with food, and most of them have reported that "the hungries are gone." Surely any physician whose patient has this type of problem can try having the patient take the T_4 with food to see if the cravings go away. Believe me, they do in almost every case. A few such patients require more T_4 because of the reduced T_4 absorption due to mixing with food, but this effect is surprisingly uncommon. Unfortunately, when someone gains 50 pounds in 5 years on 100 percent T_4 on an empty stomach, the weight does not go away readily on any regimen even if the patient feels remarkably better. A common report from such a patient looking back over a year or so has been "at least I stopped gaining on your regimen." Getting rid of food cravings by taking thyroid with food can be done by any physician. If you do this with a few patients, and it clearly works, you should be more receptive to the other ideas that are expressed in this book. My theory about this effect is that thyroid hormone contacting the stomach wall has never occurred in the evolution of the human race until we started taking oral thyroid about a century ago. It could be that the thyroid is affecting leptin and ghrelin, which are hormones produced by the stomach and which clearly have some effect in weight regulation.

TIMING OF THYROID DOSES AND SLEEP

In early 2005, a patient of mine who was following an Internet thyroid site told me that a number of individuals reported better sleep by changing their thyroid to the p.m. This reminded me of several studies published about 15 years ago in which volunteers were given IV catheters to allow easy blood drawing, and blood samples for TSH were drawn every hour over the course of 24 hours (recent example *JCEM* 93:2300, 2008). The first thing that is clear is that TSH actually varies significantly during the course of the day, further undercutting the idea that the TSH is an absolute test of thyroid function. However, the main observation is that everyone has an increase in TSH starting about 2 to 4 hours before their biological clocks say that they are going to sleep. Since TSH originates in the pituitary gland in the brain, and an increase in TSH begets an increase in thyroid hormone secretion, it appears that the body's natural rhythms call for more thyroid to be introduced into the system as we go to sleep. When I had my patients change their thyroid dosing to the evening meal, several of them found that their sleep was worse and they felt over-stimulated while trying to sleep. On their own, they figured out that it had to be the T_3, so they changed their compounded T_3 or thyroid extract capsules to breakfast, but kept their T_4 pills with the evening meal. For many of these patients, the improvement in sleep quality is remarkable. However, as in all areas of thyroid replacement, standard "cookie-cutter" approaches do not work for everyone. If the patient can take both thyroid preparations in the morning and have good sleep quality, I have them do it that way, for the convenience of once-daily dosing. Some patients have actually done better with splitting their T_4 dose between breakfast and dinner, although as physicians we were all taught that, because of the long half-life of T_4, there is no benefit in splitting doses of T_4. Any physician who is treating a patient who has a major sleep disorder with 100 percent T_4 can certainly have patients try taking their T_4 with the evening meal without worrying too much about "deviating from medical practice guidelines." Very important is that the T_4 needs to be taken 3 to 5 hours before bedtime. If taken at bedtime, it appears to have very little benefit for sleep quality.

ALLERGIES TO THYROID PILLS

Another area where any physician can make some revealing observations is concerning allergy to the thyroid pills. While this can be related to differences in excipient materials (binders and fillers) in the pills, it most often is related to the multiple dyes that are used in the color-coded systems that all the manufacturers use. For instance, the most popular single thyroid hormone dosage is probably Synthroid 0.1 mg. This contains yellow 6 and yellow 10 dyes. The 0.05 mg tablets are generally made dye-free in all the brands. If a patient on 0.1 mg of T_4 (Synthroid or other brand) says yes to questions about nasal congestion and even intermittent asthma, one can do the simple trial of giving samples of the 0.05 mg tabs and having the patient take two daily. Physicians will be very impressed by changes in their patients over 4 to 5 days if they take this approach. This maneuver results in the patient taking more thyroid pills for sure, but it often solves the fundamental problem of allergy without the expense of a steroid nasal inhaler or intermittent use of albuterol inhalers. The Synthroid brand contains such excipient materials as acacia, povidone, and talc, which are not present in the Levoxyl brand. Levothroid had been free of povidone for many years, but it has now been added in a recent reformulation of this product. Because of the presence of acacia uniquely in the Synthroid brand, if a patient continues to have nasal allergy symptoms on dye-free 0.05 mg Synthroid tablets, it is worth a trial of the Levoxyl or Levothroid brands. At this point I think that Levoxyl is the best choice because of the absence of acacia, povidone, and talc. Also, all the brand and generic T_4 preparations contain dyes in all sizes other than the 0.05 mg (50 mcg) pills. All of these dyes contain aluminum. I do not know if these dyes represent any long-term hazard to health, but my preference is to avoid aluminum by staying away from the dyes. A recent welcome addition to the T_4 field is Tirosint, a preparation that eliminates all dyes and excipient materials, save for glycerin and gelatin.

A recent observation is that many patients have adverse effects from povidone, which might be taken to mean that there is something wrong with their thyroid balance. They feel tired, have brain fog, and feel achy, often 3 to 6 hours after they take the pill in the a.m. Once this period clears, they feel very well until the following morning. Recently, I have had numerous patients who have done much better in general by switching to the Levoxyl brand. Typically, when a patient says that they "do better" on one brand than another, it is dismissed with the comment that "they are all the same." Here again, the approach should be functional. If somebody feels lousy on Synthroid or Levothroid, try having them skip the pills for a day or two and then resume. The patients who are sensitive to povidone will often report that they are remarkably better even on the first day without the pills and that the symptoms come back again as soon as they resume taking them. Think of how many patients you have seen over the years who look to be in perfect balance on Synthroid and yet still feel lousy. I have long wished a manufacturer would create T_4 pills without dyes or excipient materials, and that need has now been met by Tirosint.

CLINICAL OBSERVATIONS

A story that every physician has heard many times but has never really understood is the typical thyroid patient who presents with a low T_4, high TSH, and a strong clinical picture of hypothyroidism. This is a situation in which all of us agree on the diagnosis. When such a patient is started on T_4, he or she often experiences remarkable improvement that lasts a few months and then, on every revisit, he or she starts complaining of hypothyroid symptoms again. The standard response on the part of the physician is that "you are on thyroid and your TSH is now normal, so your symptoms can't be hypothyroid in nature. Indeed, there are a few patients, perhaps 20 percent, who continue to do extremely well on 100 percent T_4. Presumably, these individuals are good converters of T_4 to T_3, so they wind up with a favorable T_4:T_3 balance in their body tissues. However, the majority of patients (perhaps 70 to 80 percent) never feel well again on 100 percent T_4 after their initial improvement. This is the picture presented by many patients who come to me, and they almost all have remarkable improvement on addition of time-release T_3 or thyroid extract in the proper proportions. Those are simple factual observations. My theory about this may not be correct, but I believe that the answer lies in the role of TSH in stimulating the major deiodinase enzyme, which causes the conversion of T_4 to T_3 in body tissues. When first diagnosed, the high levels of TSH are maintaining near-normal T_3 levels in the tissues because of rapid conversion. As therapy with T_4 proceeds, the T_4 goes up and the TSH goes down, gradually squeezing off some of the T_4 to T_3 conversion. At a critical point, the T_3 level in tissues is suppressed below optimal and the patient has the return of symptoms. This initial response and then failure of treatment is so common that I call it the "up and down phenomenon." My belief is that the longer that 100 percent T_4 treatment proceeds, the more a T_4:T_3 imbalance is created, which will not respond to more T_4 as is usually done. The questions of the amount of T_3 and what to do with the T_4 dose in such a patient is discussed in detail later, because doing it just right is critical to getting a good result.

Every practicing endocrinologist sees patients who come through the door with a long list of complaints and are waving either printouts from the Internet or a book like mine. They report they feel poorly on T_4 and ask if the endocrinologist can treat them according to this literature. Patients coming to me report almost 100 percent rejection of those ideas and they are retold the old myth that "nobody needs T_3 because T_4 is converted to T_3 in the body." All of us physicians have a certain belief in our knowledge and are not receptive to something completely different from what we were taught. When a physician hears these challenging questions from desperate patients, he can (1) define the other M.D. as being wrong because "no studies prove what he says" or (2) allow for a slight possibility that the other M.D. might be· correct and "maybe I had better find out more about this." If any physician thoughtfully considers the observations that I have made in this chapter and matches them up with what they see in everyday practice, my belief is that there will be some realization that the teachings of the last 30 to 35 years may not be as correct as we thought.

Something that every endocrinologist sees from time to time is the patient who comes in with a distinctly low T_4 and a very high TSH (for example, from 50 to 100) and wonders why the patient's symptoms are not overwhelming. The usual physician response is that "it is surprising that you are not in a coma on a respirator with thyroid test results like this." I believe the fundamental reason for this disparity is because very high levels of TSH are intensely stimulating T_4 to T_3 conversion in peripheral tissues. The net result is that T_4 levels might be 30 percent below optimal, but the T_3 levels within tissue are being maintained at perhaps 5 percent below optimal. The addition of 100 percent T_4 to this situation increases both T_4, and at first T_3, so the patient hits a "sweet spot" a week or two into the treatment and then has a return of some of the hypothyroid symptoms even though the TSH has come down to perhaps 1 to 2. This is the precise chain of events that mandates the use of T_3 for optimal result. However, the usual physician response is "you are on thyroid and your TSH is now normal, so your symptoms can't be hypothyroid in nature." Wrong! There is practically nothing in this book more reliable and predictable than the fact that such a patient just outlined will have a beneficial response to T_3. For instance, if the patient is on 50 mcg of T_4 with good lab values, what should be done is to prescribe a time-release T_3 capsule of 0.75 mcg or 5 mg of thyroid extract in time-release form and not reduce the T_4. Considering that many physicians have given T_3 in 5 to 25 mcg doses in the past in the form of Cytomel, writing a prescription for 0.75 mcg of time-release T_3 should not be a cause of worry. Any physician who follows the above procedure will be rewarded with a happy patient.

CHAPTER 3

The TSH Myth

ONE OF the most sacrosanct teachings in all of medicine is that a TSH test is the absolute indicator of thyroid status. Since the introduction of this test in the early to mid 1970s, all physicians have been taught that a normal TSH rules out hypothyroidism. On the basis of my own experience over many years, I believe that this teaching is the biggest single mistake ever made in the entire history of medicine. Since 1985, I have followed what I would now call a functional definition of hypothyroidism in my own practice. By that I mean that if a patient comes to me with many symptoms and physical findings suggestive of hypothyroidism, I have empirically treated them even if their TSH is well within the "normal" range. In the years since 1985, I have personally started over 1,000 patients on thyroid replacement despite their never having had a high TSH value. It is true that patients with gross hypothyroidism will often present to doctors with the typical clinical picture and have a very high TSH and a low T_4—all physicians are in agreement on these patients. However, there are other factors involved in TSH regulation such that mild hypothyroidism can be masked when the TSH is normal.

The simple fact that I have violated this practice rule over a thousand times during the last 20 years or so and have a hugely successful practice with no malpractice suits in my entire history should be convincing to other physicians. In the recent literature, several studies have been published taking patients with apparent clinical hypothyroidism but normal TSH and randomizing them in clinical trials to placebo and "thyroid." The fact that all such studies conclude that thyroid hormone treatment of normal TSH patients was not beneficial is irrelevant, because they used only 100 percent T_4 and gave 3 to 4 times the appropriate dose. Doing studies in this way causes T_4 levels to go above optimum and suppresses TSH, which reduces T_4 to T_3 conversion. The net resulting T_4-T_3 balance in tissues is then unfavorable, hence the negative results. Because T_4 pills have been manufactured for many years in sizes ranging between 25 and 300 mcg, and 100 mcg may be the single most-prescribed size, several such trials have used 100 mcg, with negative results of "thyroid treatment" (Example: *BMJ* 323:891, 2001).

Because of the overdose in these trials, many people note improvement in the early weeks as proper balance is obtained and then proceed to distort T_4:T_3 balance until, at the end of the study, they are unchanged or even worse because of the treatment. I believe that the major factor which can cause a normal TSH result in a patient who actually nonetheless has hypothyroidism is the deiodinase enzyme in the pituitary gland. When a patient is clinically hypothyroid, this enzyme is activated in an attempt to maintain near-normal tissue levels of T_3 (the active hormone) despite below-optimum T_4 levels. I believe that a variety of factors, especially drugs such as Prozac, enhance the activity of that enzyme, which results in excessive amounts of T_3 being generated inside the pituitary itself, thus falsely suppressing the TSH value. This excessive activity in the pituitary appears to be reduced on empirical thyroid replacement therapy, which results frequently in elevation of the TSH value during treatment, an observation that is impossible to explain by standard wisdom in the field.

As a result of the absolute belief in the TSH number, many hypothyroid patients are assured that "it is not your thyroid." Because of depression, sleep disturbance, and lack of mental focus, such patients are often diverted to a life on antidepressants, sleeping pills, and stimulant drugs for "adult ADD." All of these treatment modalities help to some degree but they never solve the fundamental problems associated with hypothyroidism. Hence, a subpar quality of life for such individuals. In particular, the institution of antidepressant therapy in such patients becomes a frustrating dead end for the patient. The antidepressants often have very little benefit because of the underlying hypothyroidism, a fact that is well recognized in the standard practice of medicine. When frustrated patients in this category go to different physicians seeking help for their symptoms, each new physician changes them to a different antidepressant, which again usually has very little benefit. Each new physician is hesitant to stop the antidepressant treatment, although it is not working well, fearing that a subsequent major problem such as suicide will then, of course, be blamed on "stopping the antidepressant."

An empirical trial of thyroid in such a case is orders of magnitude safer than the drugs that are thrown at these patients. The way I do it is to give each patient 7 tablets of T_4 at 50 mcg and have them take ½ tablet daily. This is generally enough to close the gap between where the patient is at the start and optimum levels, with resulting improvement in energy and other symptoms. Above all, this low dose is very unlikely to close the gap and then put the T_4 level above the optimum point. My observation is that patients with a TSH in the higher end of the normal range generally need more thyroid than those in the lower part of the range. There are a few patients who can continue to feel extremely well on 25 mcg of T_4, but most of them actually experience the "up and down phenomenon." They will often report back at 2 to 3 weeks that they are much better and then report in another few weeks that it "stopped working." As a general rule, this sequence means that the patient also needs some T_3. My practice is to prescribe a time-release T_3 or thyroid extract capsule with the same amount of T_3 in order to produce a 98.5 to 1.5 T_4:T_3 ratio. For 25 mcg of T4, this means 0.375 mcg of T_3 or 2.5 mg of thyroid extract. With few exceptions, such a maneuver puts people back very quickly in the "sweet spot" and they feel much better. Despite the standard wisdom that the institution of T_3 requires the proportional reduction of T_4 dosage to avoid "toxicity," my experience is that doing time-release T_3 or thyroid extract actually increases the T_4 requirement over time, if anything. The "up and down phenomenon" is extremely common in this type of treatment. When this occurs in the type of patient just described, the remedy is to increase the T_4 and decrease T_3 or leave it unchanged. There is no simple rule to follow in such treatment and very often I find myself literally flipping a coin to decide where to go with the patient's dosage. If one elects to change the dosage of T_3 or thyroid extract, the result of doing so is usually evident in a very short period of time due to the direct action of T_3. With an adjustment of T_4, one must be cognizant that this hormone is not directly active itself and has a very long half-life, so changes in T_4 do take a number of weeks or even months before one sees the final result. Because of that, if I want to see the result of a higher T_4 dose, I typically increase the dose of T_4 by 50 percent to 100 percent for 3 to 5 days, then bring it back to a slightly higher dosage than they had before. If I think a patient needs a lower T_4 level, as often occurs in the spring due to declining seasonal needs, I have patients stop T_4 for several days and then resume it at the lower dose. Generally, speaking, the results of maneuvers like this become fairly obvious by 2 to 3 weeks.

CHAPTER 4

The Incidence of Hypothroidism

THE INCIDENCE of hypothyroidism is, in my opinion, vastly underestimated. One of the standard textbooks (*Williams Endocrinology*, 10th Edition, page 423) states that hypothyroidism affects 2 percent of adult women and 0.1 percent to 0.2 percent of adult men. Subclinical hypothyroidism, defined as a slight elevation of TSH in the presence of a normal T_4, was said to be present in 9.5 percent of individuals in a 26,000-patient study. Some other sources have given the incidence in adult women as up to 5 percent or so. My belief is that the clinical problem is probably 10 times as common as the textbooks say.

To understand this discrepancy better, let me try to explain as best I can how both sides of this argument have come to their conclusions. On the formal academic side, the belief has always been that the TSH test is an absolute indicator of underlying thyroid status. The overwhelming majority of clinical hypothyroidism is primary hypothyroidism, meaning a failure of the thyroid gland itself. There is a small subset of patients who have clinical hypothyroidism because of inadequate TSH stimulation of a normal thyroid gland, designated secondary hypothyroidism. If one does measurements of TSH in a large number of patients, the distribution will look approximately like the graph shown here.

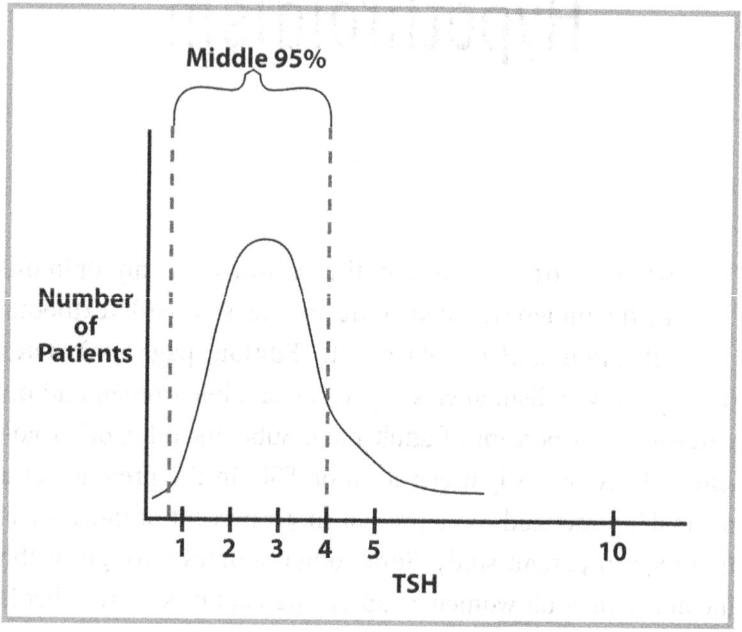

Making the fundamental assumption that hypothyroidism only affects 3 percent to 5 percent of a population distribution and that TSH is an absolute measure of thyroid function, the determination of who is normal and who is not is essentially done on the basis of chopping out the middle 95 percent of this distribution curve.

There is also the matter of "Subclinical Hypothyroidism," defined by a mildly elevated TSH and normal total T_4 or free T_4 (free T_4 measures the T_4 in serum not bound to proteins and which is, therefore, physiologically active). Many articles have been written about this condition, generally concluding that there is no evidence that treating it does any good. Once one recognizes that premenstrual syndrome (PMS), many sleep disorders, many cases of diffuse aching and stiffness, and some cases of "Adult Attention Deficit Disorder (ADD)" are related to underlying hypothyroidism, this statement that treating subclinical hypothyroidism does no good is exposed for the myth that it is. The only thing that matters is whether a patient with symptoms consistent with hypothyroidism improves or does not improve on an intelligent therapeutic trial of thyroid hormone. The fact that some distinguished academic physicians have published papers concluding that the treatment of subclinical hypothyroidism does no good does not automatically make this medical fact. In order to have normal thyroid function, one must have adequate secretion of TRH (Thyroid Releasing Hormone) from the brain stimulating the pituitary gland to release adequate TSH, which in turn stimulates the thyroid gland to release adequate thyroid hormone. In my extensive clinical experience, there are large numbers of individuals who have symptomatic hypothyroidism and respond extremely well to empirical treatment with thyroid hormone despite having TSH "in the normal range." This raises the possibility of whether large numbers of people in the population are having mild impairment of pituitary activity as they get older. Researchers have investigated such a possibility in the past by TRH stimulation testing and then measuring the TSH response to a dose of TRH. This type of testing in individual patients is expensive, has adverse effects, and is generally impractical in the office setting. The question of whether a patient has elements of both primary hypothyroidism (a problem of the thyroid gland) or secondary hypothyroidism (a problem of the pituitary gland or higher centers in the brain) is an interesting question but probably irrelevant to the care of individual thyroid patients. Unless the patient has a major problem with the pituitary gland, the only thing that matters in my opinion is whether the patient gets clearly better on thyroid hormone replacement or not. Theoretically, patients with a significant element of secondary hypothyroidism could be treated with TSH injections, but that is not a practical possibility at this time.

This brings us once again to the central focus of this book: the functional approach to hypothyroidism. If a patient has a long history of multiple symptoms and also has some physical findings suggestive of hypothyroidism, my belief is that the only thing that matters is the result of an intelligent therapeutic trial of thyroid hormone. If they are given too much thyroid or given 100 percent T_4 exclusively, many will indeed come back and report "no benefit." The physicians who would dismiss everything I have said in this chapter as "overdiagnosing hypothyroidism" are quite comfortable in prescribing antidepressants, sleeping pills, and amphetamine stimulants instead. The thing that I would like to destroy forever is the mistaken belief that a "normal" TSH takes hypothyroidism off the table as an explanation for the symptoms that patients have. I will once again state my opinion flatly, that the standard wisdom of "ruling out" hypothyroidism on the basis of a TSH result has been the biggest single mistake in the history of medicine, because it affects millions of people and results in huge over-prescribing of unnecessary and expensive drugs.

CHAPTER 5

T_3 or Not T_3 . . . That Is the Question

SINCE THE 1970s, all physicians have been taught that "nobody needs T_3 because T_4 is converted to T_3 in the body." In my own practice, I have used T_3 routinely since 1990, largely because of the observation that once patients completed the "up and down phenomenon" in their early treatment, they never felt well again unless some T_3 was added. When I decided to cross the T_3 line myself, on seeing that the T_3 hormone (Cytomel) was available in sizes of 5, 25, and 50 (5/25/50) mcg, I started by having people take 5 mcg, thinking it was a "low" dose. I very quickly found that patients in good T_4 balance were often extremely sensitive to T_3 and so, during the early 1990s my practice was to have patients cut the Cytomel 5 mcg tablet into halves or quarters. Results at that time were not consistent, but there were enough successes to make me persist despite the medicolegal risk of going against standard wisdom in the field.

The fortunate break that led to the current success that I enjoy in my practice came in 1996, when I heard a radio ad for a local compounding pharmacy indicating "we can put anything in a time-release capsule, just ask your doctor." I had fantasized about being able to conjure up T_3 time-release capsules in any dosage I wanted, but I thought it would be too expensive, especially since compounded prescriptions are often not paid for by insurance. However, I was driven to call the advertising pharmacist and ask him how much it would cost to put 100 T_3 time-release capsules into a patient's hand. The answer was "about $50" for 100 capsules and I decided to go ahead with this. In the next few years, it became clear that this was the answer for many thyroid patients who had been symptomatic for years or even decades. For some, the difference was like giving up a 20-year-old Yugo for a new BMW.

There was no support for the use of T_3 in the literature until 1999, when a study from Lithuania was published (*NEJM* 340:424, 1999). In this study, the researchers took patients on the standard T_4 treatment, randomized them to either receive a dose of T_3 or a placebo, and ultimately reported that T_3 made the patients better mentally and physically. This paper led to widespread trials of T_3 using Cytomel at two levels. Thyroid practitioners saw this as a possible answer to the question of why the huge majority of their patients who are on standard 100 percent T_4 come in complaining all the time about how they feel. It also launched a barrage of what I would characterize as "me too" studies in this country and abroad, essentially doing the same thing as the Lithuanian study.

Many academicians did trials of Cytomel in the early 2000s because of this study, most of whom are now convinced T_3 offers no benefit. The general observations here were that patients often had remarkable benefit in the first week or so on T_3, but were either worse or no better after a period of time on T_3. These practitioners figured that with Cytomel available at 5/25/50 mcg, that 5 to 10 mcg was a "low dose." Many of the leading endocrinologists in my part of the country did trials just like this, which I heard about firsthand because many of their former patients are now in my practice. This view was also enforced by the publication of numerous "me too" studies that claimed to prove that T_3 makes people worse rather than better (*JCEM* 90:805, 2005). (*JCEM* 90:266, 2005). (*AIM* 42:412, 2005).

The fundamental problem that has turned the tide against the use of T_3 is a simple matter of dose. In my extensive experience, the average daily dose of T_3 that results in sustained long-term improvement is about 1.2 mcg daily in time-release form. The empirical use of Cytomel in the early 2000s was typically done in the dose range of 5 to 25 mcg daily, in the belief that this is a "low dose" based on the fact that the Cytomel pills have been on the market since 1960 at 5/25/50 mcg. Also, based on the five to six studies that have been uniformly negative on the benefit of T_3 used in daily doses in the 6-to-25 mcg range. These studies also made the mistake of lowering T_4 by 4 mcg for each 1 mcg of T_3 given, which further exacerbates the resulting T_4:T_3 imbalance caused by too high a percentage of T_3 in the mixture.

The fundamental thing that all these researchers have completely missed is that Cytomel has been on the market at 5/25/50 mcg because of the perception that the use of T_3 would be as replacement therapy. When T_3 became available to researchers in the late 1950s, no one had the foresight to think about T_4-T_3 combinations and instead focused on the known fact that T_3 was the active hormone and might be better replacement therapy than T_4. When people with little or no intrinsic thyroid function of their own (from surgery or radioactive iodine) were replaced with T_3 totally, the typical dose requirement for those individuals to feel reasonably functional was about 75 to 100 mcg. The belief at that time that doctors would typically be prescribing 50 to 100 mcg daily led to the marketing of this pill at 5/25/50 mcg. For a variety of reasons, long-term replacement on 100 percent T_3 really does not work very well, so this use died out within a few years of the introduction of Cytomel. The fundamental reason why all this empirical use of Cytomel and T_3 studies came to the conclusion that T_3 does not help simply comes down to a matter of dose. When patients are on 100 percent T_4, most of them have a mild T_3 deficit at tissue level. When they are given even 5 mcg T_3, that gap closes very quickly and they experience immediate benefit, but the levels quickly go through the "sweet spot" and soar well above optimal levels. When dealing with physiologic hormone replacement, one has to understand that optimum benefit occurs when one reproduces the fundamental normal levels. Giving more than the required dose and going above the optimum T_3 level does not give increasing benefit, and in fact, it makes people feel worse, which was what was observed in these studies. Every 5 to 10 years, I get a patient who is taking 25 to 50 mcg of T_3 daily. They invariably show immeasurably low T_4 and TSH values, and they feel awful. They all remember feeling dramatically better at the start of T_3, peaking out after a few weeks, then feeling progressively worse as T_4 depletion occurs. I believe there has never been a patient who feels well on a regimen like this after a few months, so it mystifies me why any practitioner would prescribe it.

Optimum thyroid replacement therapy requires the establishment of the ideal T_4:T_3 ratio in the treatment. A standard practice in doing T_3 is that "1 mcg of T_3 is metabolically equivalent to 4 mcg of T_4." As a result of this teaching, which is completely fallacious, T_4 would be decreased by 20 mcg if one were to give 5 mcg of T_3. Because of this fundamentally wrong teaching and the use of too high a dose of T_3, the patients have a long-term depletion of T_4 at tissue level; this issue will be discussed in another chapter. Since the body has far more T_4 than T_3, the institution of an unbalanced T_4:T_3 regimen results in the gradual decline of T_4 tissue levels. The positive result in the Lithuanian study was due, by accident, to the fact that the study period was 5 weeks. By that time, T_4 depletion does not occur sufficiently to make people feel worse. In contrast, the more recent studies have typically been one year or so, by which time everyone is terribly T_4-depleted and thus registers a negative response to the institution of T_3.

A few years ago, a representative from the pharmaceutical company that makes Cytomel called on me and said that the company was considering making Cytomel into time-release capsules. I suspect that idea is now completely in limbo because of the overwhelming literature evidence that T_3 is not helpful. Unless I have a unique ability to induce placebo responses in many hundreds of patients over many years, T_3 is in fact critical for treatment of hypothyroidism. I explained to this representative how the 5/25/50 mcg tablets represented extreme overdosage. If they could make time-release capsules or pills at significantly lower cost than the current individually compounded prescriptions, this would be a huge advance in thyroid treatment. I suspect that since all leaders in this field believe that T_3 is of no use, this project is probably buried. In my opinion, what are necessary are 0.1/0.3/0.5/1.0 mcg capsules. In between dosages could then be given combining two or three of the manufactured dosages. One thing I can guarantee is that if Cytomel is ever made in time-release capsules of 5/25/50 mcg, this will be a total failure.

CHAPTER 6

The T_2 Question

ONE OF the things that every experienced thyroid physician has seen is an older hypothyroid patient who has seen multiple physicians and notes that "the only time I felt great is when I was switched to Armour." (Armour is the extract of porcine thyroid glands, which has been used for thyroid replacement therapy for over a century.) The usual observation is that the benefit of Armour lasts for a few weeks to a few months and then the patient feels as poorly as before. Testing at that point will often show a relatively low TSH, so the answer is clearly not to give more Armour. I believe that the brief period of well-being occurs because of the mixture present in the natural product and that the fading of the result occurs because of gradual tissue T_4 depletion due to the 80:20 T_4:T_3 nature of Armour.

This was a question that had always intrigued me, since I had heard this from a number of patients coming to me. As a result, I started in 2001 to have my compounding pharmacist put thyroid extract powder into time-release capsules, and I switched people from time-release T_3 capsules to time-release thyroid extract capsules with the same amount of T_3 as before. There was no doubt in my mind that the huge majority of patients were distinctly better on thyroid extract even though their overall T_4 and T_3 doses were the same as before. Because of the success in making this transition that I had observed in many patients, my practice now has about 90 percent of the patients taking thyroid extract rather than pure T_3. For a variety of reasons, some people prefer not to be taking the natural pig thyroid extract, but they do almost as well on T_3.

The major difference I have observed on switching people from T_3 to thyroid extract is better mental function. The special benefit of using thyroid extract rather than pure synthetics is probably the presence of a breakdown product (T_2) in the natural product. If there is anything to the rumor that T_2 can enhance weight loss, it is not evident in my experience, but the amount of T_2 in the extract that I am giving is very low. There is no way to know what would happen if T_2 were available and dosages of it could be compounded into a thyroid extract capsule. For those who are squeamish about pig thyroid, one could use time-release capsules of synthetic T_3 and T_2. To be more precise, one must realize that there are three different T_2 isomers (molecular variants) due to the different positions of the iodine atoms, as shown on the following page.

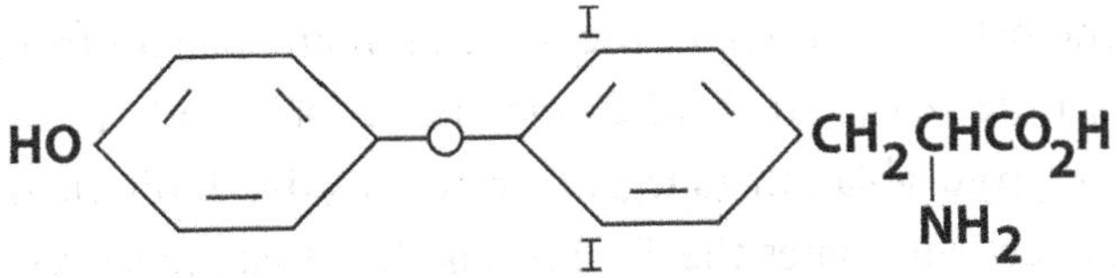

3, 5

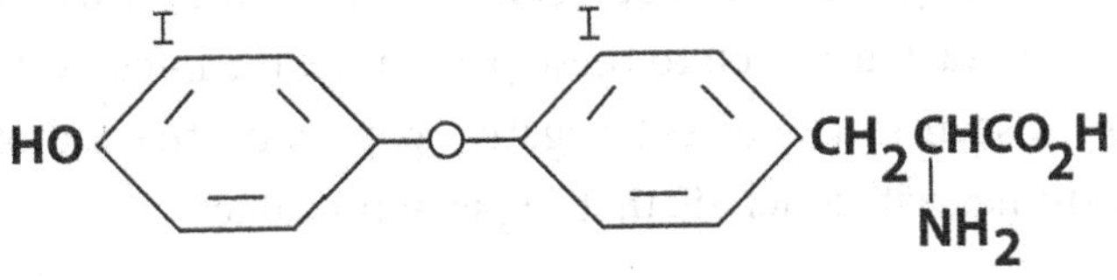

3, 3′

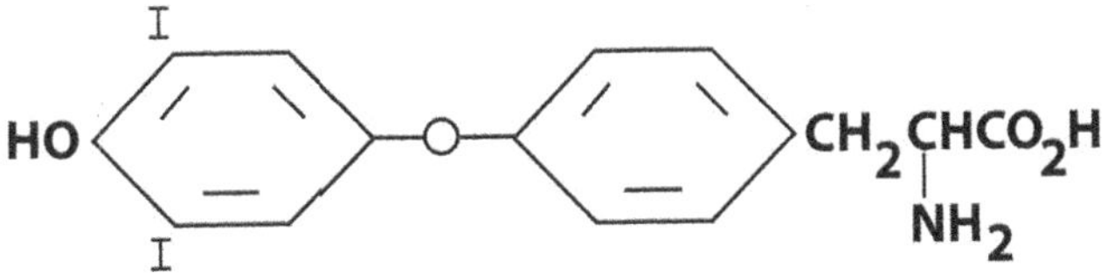

3′ 5′

It appears that the active T_2 is the 3, 5 isomer.

The patients who have the most dramatic benefit from the use of time-release thyroid extract are those who have undergone thyroid ablation (surgery or radioactive iodine), which completely eliminates the T_3, T_2's, and T_1's that are secreted by the normal gland. Every physician that does this knows that such patients given 100 percent T_4 almost always feel miserable ever after. The improvement in thyroid ablation patients given the type of regimen that I have outlined above is so dramatic and so universal that it is high time that the academic leaders in this field recognize it. Of course, if they do studies where T_3 or thyroid extract are given to these patients in the huge overdose range as seen in the recent negative papers on the use of T_3, their studies will conclude that "T_3 is of no value."

CHAPTER 7

T_4 DEPLETION

THE CONCEPT of T_4 depletion over time on various thyroid regimens is key in understanding many of the things that physicians observe in their practices every day and is also crucial to understanding what is published in the standard medical literature. An old teaching that continues to be followed to this present day is that 1 mcg of T_3 is metabolically equivalent to 4 mcg of T_4, so that if a patient has good laboratory numbers on a given dose of T_4, the physician should subtract 4 mcg of T_4 for each 1 mcg of T_3 to be given. Out of curiosity, I tried backtracking through a number of papers on this subject trying to find out the origin of this teaching. It ended with a reference to the British Formulary simply stating that 1 mcg of T_3 equals 4 mcg of T_4. To me, this is like saying if you want to reduce meat consumption by one pound per week, you should substitute four bananas. It does not compute! It is my contention that many of the negative results that physicians have seen with T_3 and also see in medical journals reporting negatively on T_3 are related to T_4 depletion over time. In my own extensive practice over the past 15 years or so, patients coming in on a good T_4 dose are usually about the same or slightly higher on their T_4 dose a year later, after T_3 or thyroid extract is added, and they are still doing very well with normal laboratory values.

The major factor leading to all the negative T_3 literature is the use of too much T_3. As explained elsewhere, the fact that Cytomel has been on the market for 50 years or so in sizes of 5/25/50 mcg really has no relevance to the needs of the individual patient being given a T_4:T_3 regimen. The negative studies on T_3 used daily doses of 6 to 25 mcg, which is 10 to 20 times the appropriate dose. In my successful practice, the average T_3 dose is around 1.2 mcg daily. The human thyroid probably secretes about a 95:5 T_4:T_3 mixture into the system daily. When such a patient is given a regimen with 80:20 or 70:30 T_4:$T_{3,}$ as has occurred in many of these studies, they will gradually desaturate T_4 in the peripheral tissues and then the whole metabolic effect fails. Since there is so much more T_4 in the body than T_3, this T_4 depletion takes some time, so that the patient typically feels very well for a short period of time before eventually winding up feeling worse than before. When the patient is evaluated at the end of a typical one-year study and reports "worse than ever," the researchers then report "T_3 made the patient worse." The fact that the 1999 Lithuanian study reported a benefit from T_3 was due to the fact that this was a five-week study so that there was not a significant amount of T_4 depletion by that time. I guarantee that if the same protocol had been extended to a study of 12 to 15 weeks, the result would have been negative just as the later papers on the subject were.

Following the 1999 report indicating benefit from T_3, many of the leading academic physicians in my area decided to try

T_3. Given the 5/25/50 mcg sizes of Cytomel, they reasoned that 5/10/15 mcg of T_3 daily would be a "low dose." There is also the regimen popularized by Dr. Ridha Arem (*The Thyroid Solution*, Ballantine Books, 1999), who advocates a regimen using 5 mcg Cytomel two or three times daily. What happens in virtually every case is that the T_3 levels hit the "sweet spot" in just a day or two and the patient feels fantastically better, but this fades very rapidly after a week or two. This is because the T_3 dose is so high that it hits the optimum point very quickly and then goes above the optimum point, and you do not get more and more benefit by giving more and more of a physiologic hormone. Time and time again, physicians will notice that patients have many of the same symptoms above the optimum point as they had when they were below. When patients are given 5 or 10 mcg of Cytomel and report back to their physicians in 3 months or so, their verdict is usually "worse than ever." When they ask why it was that they felt wonderful the first week, it is dismissed as a "placebo effect." It is not a placebo effect. The optimum dose of T_3 per day for most patients is on the order of 1.2 mcg and giving more never gives more benefit.

In summary, then, the T_4 reduction at the start of treatment due to the mistaken assumption that 1 mcg T_3 equals 4 mcg $T_{4,}$ along with the use of a T_4:T_3 regimen too heavily weighted toward $T_{3,}$ causes T_4 depletion over time, thus explaining the initial benefit and the ultimate lack of benefit.

CHAPTER 8

The PMS-Thyroid Connection

IN 1986, Brayshaw and Brayshaw published a letter in the *New England Journal of Medicine* (*NEJM* 315:1486, 1986). In that letter, they laid out a clinical trial involving the use of thyroid hormone for the symptoms of premenstrual syndrome (PMS). They basically decided to start 34 women in their practice who had normal thyroid tests and were also experiencing severe PMS on 25 mcg of T4, and their plan was to increase to 50 mcg the second month, 75 mcg the third month, and so on. During the first month, all 34 reported remarkable improvement and so the authors rushed into print with this letter, no doubt to ensure their claim to being first in this area. However, nothing was ever heard from them again. A few years later around 1990, I was attending a lecture by one of the Boston academic thyroid specialists when he was asked about thyroid and PMS by a member of the audience. His reply was that the editors of the Journal should never have allowed that letter to be published because it has been disproven and makes no sense. What happened was that PMS returned in the second month on 50 mcg and eventually a number of patients developed symptoms of hyperthyroidism and the whole trial fell apart.

Because this letter had gotten into print, PMS sufferers were going to their doctors in droves asking for the new miracle treatment. Of course, their doctors said they had been checked for hypothyroidism and that "your tests are within normal limits." Because of the Brayshaw letter, reports on two major academic studies of the PMS-thyroid question were published in the early 1990s (*JCEM* 70:1108, 1990; *JCEM* 76:671, 1993). Basically, these studies used larger numbers of subjects, stratified them into groups with comparable characteristics, and then randomized them to receive "thyroid or placebo." Both of these studies concluded that PMS and hypothyroidism have little or nothing to do with each other and the subject has been buried since then. These are further examples of classic "triple blind" studies, since they gave patients about a 4-fold overdose of T_4 (100 mcg). Here again, patients with clinical hypothyroidism and normal TSH have dose requirements of approximately 25 mcg, so giving them a trial on 100 mcg of T_4 is bound to end with the patient feeling worse, if anything, because they have extended beyond the optimum point, thereby enhancing the resulting T_4:T_3 imbalance. Many journal articles and book chapters have been written about PMS without the word "thyroid" appearing anywhere therein. I will state categorically that premenstrual syndrome is most fundamentally a thyroid problem, although the actual mechanism is probably the thyroid effect on ovarian progesterone production.

The patients that I start on thyroid and manage on the mixed T_4-T_3 regimen that I use generally have major improvement in PMS. Several observations made by my smart and empowered patients have further refined the treatment of PMS. One of my patients decided that, because her fatigue increased as part of PMS (as it usually does), that she should take more of her "energy pill" (T_4) and noted that this had a remarkable benefit. Another patient of mine had stomach discomfort on the time-release capsules, and so I was giving her T_3 in a skin cream, which is applied by a tuberculin syringe at 0.1 cc daily. One day, during a bad PMS cycle, she noted that she felt wonderful. She then realized that she had forgotten to apply her T_3 cream that morning. So now, my fine-tuning of thyroid with respect to PMS is to have women increase their T_4 pills about 10 to 20 percent at start of PMS and stop or reduce the T_3 or thyroid extract. It is almost as if the various factors involved in PMS cause a heightened T_4 to T_3 conversion, resulting in a lower T_4 and higher T_3 than optimal. For many patients, this type of manipulation has been almost miraculous.

There is a body of literature that says that PMS responds to SSRI (selective serotonin reuptake inhibitor) antidepressant drugs such as Prozac, but I strongly suspect that the modest effect of these drugs has been overblown by academic studies funded by drug company interests. Just recently, I heard another radio ad soliciting patients to take part in a study on a new drug for PMS at one of Boston's academic hospitals. The typical story is that a drug company comes up with a newly patented, expensive drug that perhaps has some benefit for this condition. The drug company then funds a study in which the academic experts running the study somehow lose their objectivity and are sent around the country to preach the virtues of this drug to local physicians. When, coincidentally, Prozac (fluoxetine) was coming to the end of its patent a few years ago, the company launched a major drive in pushing this drug in the treatment of PMS. They put a new trade name on fluoxetine, calling it "Serafem." The obvious reason was to persuade women to specifically request this drug from their physicians. If there was any reluctance to take Prozac because of its status as a "psychiatric drug," the new name Serafem sounded nicer, having to do with women's health. Elaborate classification schemes were outlined for different types of PMS and scales for rating the severity of a variety of symptoms adding up to a PMS score were in vogue at the time. They even came up with a new name for PMS, PMDD (Premenstrual Dysphoric Disorder). All this to me was meant to make this condition seem incredibly complex and suggest to prescription-writing physicians that their PMDD problems would go away if they simply affixed their signature to a prescription for Prozac or Serafem. Thyroid treatment works like a charm—take it from me.

CHAPTER 9

Thyroid and Pregnancy

PERHAPS NOWHERE in the various topics discussed in this book is the role of thyroid more important than it is in pregnancy. It has long been a given that untreated hypothyroidism is clearly cause for infertility, miscarriage, and premature delivery, a conclusion which is universally accepted. I believed as long as 25 to 30 years ago that thyroid demand clearly increased in the course of a pregnancy, and consequently it has been my policy through my entire career to periodically raise thyroid doses in pregnancy. This was especially evident if a pregnancy was proceeding into the fall and winter, where the increased seasonal need amplified the increased thyroid need of the ongoing pregnancy. Routinely, in the fall and winter, women in various stages of pregnancy would report that they had been doing extremely well until the last 2 to 3 weeks, but now felt awful. Routinely, in a situation like that, I give the patients a "jump start" with a 25 to 50 percent increase in the T_4 dose for 3 to 4 days; I then restart them on a dose perhaps 10 percent higher than the original. This almost always results in a dramatic improvement in the overall situation within 1 to 2 weeks.

The increasing thyroid need during a pregnancy that I felt was self-evident for many years has recently been formalized by an important study (*NEJM* 351:241, 2004). However, these researchers made the typical assumption that advancing thyroid needs during a pregnancy would be announced by rising TSH levels. My belief is that increasing thyroid on a functional basis is the way to go; subsequent improvement on increase is the ultimate test of whether this is right or not. Increasing thyroid dosages during a pregnancy when the TSH is well within normal has always sent medical-legal shivers down my spine, but I have never had a significant problem occur because of overdose during a pregnancy. There have been many studies published that link the thyroid status of the mother in the first 2 months of pregnancy to the subsequent neuropsychiatric development of their children. Our Italian colleagues have recently found that there is a higher incidence of ADHD (attention-deficit hyperactivity disorder) in children of patients from low-iodine areas or who showed frank thyroid abnormalities during the pregnancy (*JCEM* 89:6054, 04). This is strictly anecdotal, but my observation after many years of treating women with increasing doses of thyroid during the pregnancy is that their children's neuropsychiatric development has been excellent virtually across the board.

One of the many observations during a pregnancy is the occurrence of acid reflux. The standard teaching in this field for many years has been that the high levels of progesterone in a pregnancy reduce the tone of the lower esophageal sphincter muscle, thus allowing the normal stomach acid to wash up the esophagus. The pressure from the pregnancy on the stomach is also deemed to be a contributing factor. What I have seen many times over in my career is that the women who are falling behind in regards to their thyroid needs during the pregnancy would come in complaining of fatigue and increasing acid reflux. Our general response to acid reflux is to encourage the frequent use of Tums or Rolaids, to relieve symptoms, protect the surface of the esophagus, and incidentally, to provide more calcium for the fetus. However, the increase in thyroid I routinely give in such situations usually results in dramatic resolution of acid reflux.

Many women with recurrent problems of infertility, miscarriage, and prematurity have been studied with respect to their status of thyroid antibodies (the presence of thyroglobulin and thyroid peroxidase antibodies indicates an autoimmune process affecting the thyroid gland). Numerous studies (example, *Fertility and Sterility* 71:843, 1999) have found a relationship between the presence of thyroid antibodies and a higher risk of these obstetrical problems in comparison to women who are negative for antibodies. For the most part, since they generally find the TSH values the same in both the antibody-positive and antibody-negative groups, the conclusion has been that thyroid function has nothing to do with these problems and it is perhaps some type of autoimmune phenomenon that is the cause. Here again, it has been believed that, because the TSH in one group of patients was the same as in the other group, this means thyroid hormone levels were not involved.

In my experience, many women empirically treated with thyroid in the face of a normal TSH overcame prior infertility problems and had wonderful full-term pregnancies. While medical science has become very good at saving premature babies, the emotional and financial cost of doing this is incredible. Given that it is very clear that thyroid needs go up in a pregnancy, I have long thought empirical treatment with 25 to 50 mcg of T_4 even in euthyroid pregnancies (pregnancies where thyroid tests are within normal limits) would probably result in great benefit. Because of the heightened medicolegal tensions felt by physicians in dealing with pregnant women, my thought for many years has been that this study would never be done. However, just such a study was recently reported from Italy (*JCEM* 91:2587, 2006). In this study, patients with histories of miscarriage and premature delivery and positive thyroid antibodies were randomized to receive placebo or 25 to 50 mcg of T_4. The treatment with T_4 was clearly shown to reduce miscarriage and prematurity to control levels. I feel that such treatment is cheap, simple, and safe and would greatly reduce the burdens of miscarriage and premature birth. However, despite this wonderful study from Italy, I doubt this will become standard practice in this country because of the medicolegal risk to the physician, in case anything should go wrong. Even I have feared to tread in this area. But we should.

Another area of immense importance is the thyroid status of the mother in the first 2 months or so of pregnancy. It is very clear that much of the important development of the brain and other neural structures is occurring at this time in the pregnancy and is very much dependent on the thyroid environment provided by the mother. There have been several studies indicating that the lower the TSH of the mother in early pregnancy, the better the neuropsychiatric development of the children. I believe that a sizable fraction of the infertility treatments that are done in this country basically serve to overcome minor ovulation, implantation, and progesterone production problems in hypothyroid women. The ovulation-stimulating drugs used in such treatment can overcome minor deficits related to underlying hypothyroidism. However, utilizing this treatment alone results in a situation in which the neuropsychiatric development of the child in the first 2 months will occur in a hypothyroid environment. Also, as the pregnancy proceeds, a mild thyroid deficit will grow. In general, I have very frequently had patients come to me with a history of multiple miscarriages, primarily in the late fall. I once read a tongue-in-cheek article that suggested late-fall prevalence of miscarriage was related to the increased conception rate in couples on vacation at the end of the summer, so the pregnancies would be at 3 months around November. However, I believe that the explanation for this phenomenon is that huge numbers of women in the population are borderline in their thyroid function, and the reduced demands of the warmer weather (and possibly the sunlight) optimizes their reproductive function at the very end of the warmest months, that is, August. By the second to the third month of the pregnancy, the fetal thyroid has essentially taken over, and the thyroid metabolism of the mother and fetus are more or less isolated from each other. Hence, if the mother becomes somewhat deficient later in a pregnancy, the fetus will probably do just fine and the mother will simply have fatigue and increased acid reflux.

An observation that has always intrigued me is that I have never seen a case of postpartum depression in any woman that I have ever managed thyroid-wise during a pregnancy. A psychiatrist at my hospital wrote a book on postpartum depression about 10 years ago and, in its 400-plus pages, the word "thyroid" never appeared. The usual professional approach to this problem centers on the use of antidepressant drugs, which is tragic for our patients. I believe that postpartum depression results from a thyroid tissue gap that has opened up because of the prolonged increased demands of the pregnancy. The fact that these patients do not announce the thyroid nature of their symptoms by having an elevated TSH test is again the fundamental problem. There are so many hormonal changes going on through a pregnancy and postpartum that I believe the TSH result is virtually irrelevant. Many of the children born to my patients exhibit early signs of superb mental and physical development, and I think that it is time that such benefits be extended to other patients as well.

CHAPTER 10

Thyroid and Depression

DEPRESSION IS very often a major component of the picture of hypothyroidism. This connection has long been recognized in the standard medical literature, although I believe the extent of the relationship is vastly underappreciated due to the belief that only depressed patients who are hypothyroid will show a TSH over the "upper limits of normal." Indeed, the history of unsuccessful treatment with numerous antidepressants of different types in and of itself strongly implies underlying hypothyroidism.

If a patient comes to me with a good clinical picture of hypothyroidism with a significant component of depression, my policy is to try them on thyroid alone. Once the antidepressant bridge is crossed, the clinical picture is muddied, so that it is difficult or impossible to decide which component of treatment is causing the good or bad things that are happening. Much more common in terms of the patients that I see are those who have indeed been on multiple antidepressants, none of which have ever worked. Since thyroid replacement therapy is simply adding physiologic amounts of hormones that are already present in the body, it is compatible with any kind of treatment. Therefore, what I do is have patients continue whatever antidepressant that they are on so that subsequent changes can indeed be attributed to the thyroid treatment. Depression is often worse in the fall or winter, so if I have a good clinical response to thyroid, I have the patient continue their antidepressant until the spring. It would not surprise me at all if we eventually find that this seasonal depressive effect has a great deal to do with sunlight exposure and the subsequent effect on Vitamin D metabolism.

An observation that I have made many times over during my career is that the institution of Prozac appears to artificially suppress TSH. Here is a composite typical scenario that many physicians can relate to and which verifies this suppression of TSH in their own practices. A woman in her early 40s comes to see the physician and relates how she has lost interest in all her pursuits, is tired all the time, feels down, and has very poor sleep. Most physicians hearing such a story will think hypothyroidism versus depression. If the lab results are well within normal, for example, T_4 is 9 and TSH is 2, the standard practice is to "rule out" hypothyroidism and diagnose depression. If such a patient is subsequently started on Prozac, there is often a significant improvement over the first couple of months and then it "stops working." What I suggest to the physician in a case like this is to check the thyroid tests after a period on Prozac. In this particular case, I predict that you will find the T_4 significantly lower, for example, at 6, and the TSH also significantly lower, for example, at 0.5. The standard take on this scenario would be that the patient is moving toward hyperthyroidism because of the lower TSH, but in that case the lower T_4 would not coincide. My belief is that what happens is that the Prozac stimulates the major deiodinase enzyme and one has an increase in T_4 to T_3 conversion in peripheral tissues and in the pituitary gland itself. The peripheral conversion gives a fast benefit in terms of mood and also contributes to the common side effect of feeling "hyper" for the first few weeks. The increased T_4 to T_3 conversion in the pituitary suppresses the TSH secretion by increasing T_3 in the pituitary, essentially setting the thyroid thermostat lower. The peripheral generation of T_3 gradually gets reduced over a few months due to depletion of the T_4 in the tissues, and the reduction in TSH also tends to reduce peripheral T_4 to T_3 conversion.

As I have written elsewhere in this book, the introduction of Cytomel (T_3) around 1960 as thyroid replacement therapy very quickly died out as it became clear that this is not good long-term replacement therapy. In the decades between then and now, most of the T_3 use has been by psychiatrists because of the empirical observation that T_3 often helps to treat depression. Historically, the typical picture has been the use of adequate dosage of an antidepressant for an adequate period of time with little or no clinical result, in which case the introduction of T_3 is sometimes very helpful. However, the psychiatrists have been even worse than the endocrinologists in terms of figuring out the proper dosage. In a recent study on the effect of T_3 on depression (*JCEM* 89:6271, 2004), the protocol was to treat a number of consecutive patients diagnosed with major depression with paroxetine (Paxil), but study the effect of supplemental T_3 (adjunctive therapy) on the therapeutic outcome. The study group was divided into "low-dose" T_3 versus "high-dose" T_3. The "low dose" in this study of T_3 was 25 mcg and the "high dose" was 50 mcg. Here again, the leaders in this field have fallen victim to the fact that the Cytomel pills are produced in sizes of 5/25/50 mcg. The simple fact is that even 5 mcg of T_3 is simply too much for any human being. There are many physicians reading this that would probably say they remember seeing a patient who was taking 50 mcg of Cytomel and did not appear to be "hyper" at all. What I would say to that is to check their thyroid function tests and I guarantee that you will see a very low T_4 as well as a TSH of zero. These people are terribly T_4 depleted, thus allowing them to tolerate huge overdoses of T_3 without manifesting symptoms of hyperthyroidism. However, this is not a normal physiology and the overall results are terrible. This study of the effect of T_3 on the treatment of depression is absolutely meaningless because of the 20- to 30-fold overdose of T_3.

I believe that this relationship between thyroid and depression has become a "black hole" into which many unfortunate patients have fallen. First, they are "ruled out" in regard to hypothyroidism by a normal TSH, and then their TSH is further artificially suppressed by the antidepressant drugs that do not work because of the underlying hypothyroidism. With a low TSH, no physician wants to start them on thyroid, and the physician is also very reluctant to stop the ineffective antidepressant, because of fear of being blamed for a subsequent disaster such as suicide. I am not saying that there is never a use for antidepressant drugs, but the current scene is certainly conducive to the sale of newer and more expensive patented antidepressants.

CHAPTER 11

Cardiac Manifestations of Hypothyroidism

IN MY clinical experience, I have found that rapid cardiac arrhythmia and congestive heart failure are two major areas of interest in cardiology where the effect of hypothyroidism is widely under-appreciated due to the complete reliance on blood test results in defining hypothyroidism.

CARDIAC ARRHYTHMIAS

A very common clinical picture seen in young women is a syndrome called mitral valve prolapse (MVP). Patients with this condition typically have a history of sudden onset of rapid heartbeat, which is unprovoked by physical exertion or emotional stress and resolves spontaneously. In some cases, the rapid heartbeat may persist for hours, which generally brings the patient to medical attention. In such cases, a routine electrocardiogram would show that the rapid rhythm originates in the atrium and travels down the normal pathways, a condition generally labeled as paroxysmal atrial tachycardia (PAT). Since PAT is often observed along with mitral valve prolapse, they are believed to be related to each other. A cardiac ultrasound is typically done as well and will often reveal a backward bulge of the mitral valve, which denoted the diagnosis of MVP. While this condition is very distressing to patients, it is not of overwhelming medical importance so it is usually treated very conservatively (such as with beta-blocker drugs to slow the ventricular response).

Women with MVP will usually also exhibit symptoms compatible with hypothyroidism such as fatigue, PMS, sleep disturbance, and irregular periods. With great trepidation a number of years ago, I started giving such patients a trial with 25 mcg of T_4. I knew that if such a patient appeared in the emergency room a few days later with a rapid heartbeat, the physician would jump to the conclusion that the T_4 brought on the rapid heartbeat. However, I have never seen this happen, and in fact, the runs of rapid heartbeat often cease upon thyroid treatment. I believe this is due to the fact that the prolapsed valve seen in MVP is a result of a malfunction of the papillary muscles, which anchor the valves. The failure of these muscles allows the valve leafs to go backward past their ordinary position, leading to the prolapse. As mentioned earlier, hypothyroidism enhances of activity of the deiodinase enzyme, which is present in cardiac muscle cells. I believe that this sets up a condition where above-normal T_3 within cardiac muscle cells causes the electrical irritability that triggers the rapid runs seen in MVP. Therefore, treatment with T_4 reduces activity of the deiodinase enzyme, while also reducing the amount of T_3 within the cardiac muscle cells.

Another common scenario in cardiology related to hypothyroidism is the common arrhythmia known as atrial fibrillation. When an older patient comes to an emergency room with sudden onset of rapid, irregular rhythm, they are often found to be in atrial fibrillation. In such cases, the physician will likely order thyroid function tests. Atrial fibrillation is often caused by an overactive thyroid and is a fairly common sign of hyperthyroidism in older patients. However, as all cardiologists are aware, many older patients may exhibit signs of atrial fibrillation but not appear to be clinically hyperthyroid at all because they have T_4 and T_3 levels at the low end of normal. Assuming that the patient's zero TSH value is not due to pituitary dysfunction, this combination of tests presents a dilemma to physicians who believe that blood tests are a definitive test for thyroid function. My belief is that these patients are, in fact, somewhat hypothyroid and that the low TSH is actually related to intense T_4 to T_3 conversion within the pituitary gland itself, which falsely suppresses the TSH. Although I have not personally treated such a patient, my belief is that a conservative treatment with T_4 would help the patient feel much better and would raise their chances of remaining in normal rhythm after they are converted to it (usually by cardioversion, an electrical shock applied to the chest under anesthesia).

CONGESTIVE HEART FAILURE

Another major area of cardiology is that of congestive heart failure, which is a frequent cause of death and disability. Congestive heart failure is marked by a low pump output by the heart, specifically an output that does not increase with an increase in heart rate. This results in poor exercise capacity and rapid onset of shortness of breath upon exertion. Anything that impairs the pump function of the heart (such as myocardial infarction or viral myocarditis) can cause this condition. In order to have normal cardiac output, the cardiac muscle must contract strongly to eject a portion of blood. It must then relax quickly to allow the filling of the left ventricle before the next electrical wave causes the ventricle to contract again. If the cardiac muscle is damaged by prior myocardial infarctions or a number of other diseases, it is unable to contract strongly enough to pump blood adequately, a condition known as systolic dysfunction. This is easy to measure and identify by using a cardiac ultrasound, which reports the ejection fraction or EF (the proportion of blood in the ventricle that has been pumped out to the body on that stroke). A very strong and healthy heart might have an EF of 60 percent to 70 percent while a badly damaged heart might only have an EF of 15 percent to 20 percent.

Thyroid function does not play a major role in systolic dysfunction. However, another type of dysfunction called diastolic dysfunction does seem to be impacted by thyroid function. Diastolic dysfunction is a condition that is not yet fully understood. In fact, it is so difficult to define this condition using the usual diagnostic procedures that the cardiologists often label it as congestive heart failure with normal ejection fraction. As explained earlier, the cardiac muscle must be able to relax quickly after contracting to squeeze blood out to the body. However, for reasons that are still unknown, patients with diastolic dysfunction have heart muscles that relax too slowly, resulting in inadequate filling of the left ventricle. In such cases, even a strong contraction would not pump the increased blood flow necessary to sustain physical activity. Over the years, I have come across a number of older patients who have come to me overdosed with thyroid (specifically T_3) and show no manifestations of congestive heart failure despite very high heart rates. In particular, I can recall a woman in her 50s who was on a regimen that included 195 mcg of T_3! She had very high blood pressure and her heart rate was 140, with minimal shortness of breath to indicate failure. Anyone with the slightest degree of diastolic dysfunction at such a high heart rate would drop their cardiac output so low that they would probably die quickly due to congestive heart failure. At very high heart rates, the left ventricle does not have time to fill, so even with a strong contraction, cardiac output drops because of much lower flow per beat. In other words, a patient who has adequate blood flow at this heart rate has demonstrated complete absence of diastolic dysfunction, presumably related to the T_3.

This example has led me to believe that at least some diastolic dysfunction is related to underlying thyroid problems. Recall, for instance, the classic presentation of hypothyroidism in which a physician can elicit slow relaxation of the ankle reflexes. The calf muscle will contract normally on tapping the Achilles tendon, but the contracted muscle relaxes very slowly, leading to the classic "hung-up" ankle reflex. If this can occur in the calf muscle with hypothyroid patients, it is likely that the cardiac muscle relaxation may also be adversely affected by hypothyroidism. The conventional reaction to this assumption would be that as long as the tests are in the normal range, the patient cannot possible have hypothyroidism. In the functional approach to hypothyroidism that I advocate, what is more relevant is whether a patient with diastolic dysfunction is being treated with T_3. My speculation would be that elderly patients who have been treated with Armour for decades would be extremely unlikely to ever show diastolic dysfunction. However, this does not mean that I would necessarily advocate T_3 treatment for older patients with diastolic dysfunction. These are fragile patients who can easily have major cardiac disasters happen at any time, and if they are being treated with T_3, the thyroid treatment would most likely be blamed for the disaster. On the other hand, if an accurate and reliable measure of diastolic dysfunction can be developed, it would be possible to establish the diastolic function in a patient who has been documented to have hypothyroidism and then see if the diastolic dysfunction eventually improves on treatment of the hypothyroidism. One could also measure diastolic function in large numbers of older people who have been on the standard 100 percent T_4 treatment. Additionally, such measurements could be taken on people at any age diagnosed as having hypothyroidism and compared to the normal ranges for that age.

CHAPTER 12

The Hypothyroidism-Fibromyalgia Connection

FIBROMYALGIA IS a commonly diagnosed condition characterized by widespread musculoskeletal pain and aching, sleep problems, and chronic fatigue. It is diagnosed almost exclusively in young to middle-aged females and is often accompanied by irritable bowel syndrome (alternating constipation and diarrhea) and menstrual disorders. The overlap in the symptoms of fibromyalgia with those of hypothyroidism is staggering—both conditions are characterized by fatigue, brain fog, muscular aches, and sleep disturbance.

There are currently no tests or biopsy findings to definitively diagnose fibromyalgia. Because of the prominence of sleep disturbance, a common treatment over the years has been amitriptyline, a sedating antidepressant drug which does provide some benefit. However, the benefit is often accompanied by fatigue persisting into the next day and weight gain. It is important to note that symptoms also seem to improve with moderate exercise and warmer weather. As is often the case, this common but mysterious illness has spawned an expensive prescription drug (Lyrica), which may have some modest benefit in alleviating symptoms.

As is often the case, academic specialists believe that, because there is no obvious difference in TSH values for patients with fibromyalgia, hypothyroidism cannot possibly be involved. Yet, in my experience, every patient I have seen who has been diagnosed with fibromyalgia has improved with thyroid hormone—some very significantly. I cannot say that any single patient was ever completely cured of their fibromyalgia symptoms, but all have improved enough to want to stay on thyroid hormone. When you examine the clinical manifestations of fibromyalgia and the patient group that is most affected by this condition, it is hard to deny the similarities with hypothyroidism. My general policy over the years has been to see how far a patient will improve once I optimize their thyroid treatment. When I feel I have gone as far as I can with thyroid treatment, I empirically try other remedies which have been reputed to have some success such as magnesium-malic acid, MSM,and SAMe. Overall, I am quite convinced that intelligent treatment with thyroid hormone is an important part of the answer to alleviating fibromyalgia.

CHAPTER 13

Susceptibility to Motion Sickness and Hypothyroidism

I BELIEVE THERE is a strong connection between hypothyroidism and sensitivity to motion sickness. One of my most frequent types of new patients are individuals who believe they have hypothyroidism after reading about the manifestations of this disease and matching them up with their own symptoms. Such patients are routinely told that they cannot have hypothyroidism because they have normal TSH test results. Even so, these patients often come to physicians with numerous complaints, all of which are consistent with hypothyroidism (such as loss of the outer eyebrows, some enlargement of the thyroid gland, and slowing of the ankle reflexes)—in other words, all the clinical manifestations necessary to make the diagnosis of hypothyroidism. When I ask about their susceptibility to motion sickness, they usually respond with amazement that I somehow knew they experience motion sickness. It is almost as though they are all reading from the same prepared statement. Nearly all of these patients explain that they are okay when driving but cannot ride in the back seat or read when in the car. These are patients who subsequently improve dramatically with empirical thyroid treatment. While symptoms like sleep disturbance often improve on the first day of thyroid replacement, improvement in susceptibility to motion sickness is a longer-term manifestation of treatment.

In trying to understand this association, I theorize that the balance center in the inner ear is adversely affected by hypothyroidism, causing frequent motion sickness. Such patients often complain of frequent episodes of vertigo, typically upon getting up in the morning or sometimes when standing after lying down for a long period of time. I can only say that patients that I have treated for years have noticed significant improvement or complete relief from this symptomatology. This is yet another example of how thyroid balance affects virtually every function in the body to some degree.

CHAPTER 14

Effect of Timing of Thyroid Dosage on Weight and Sleep

As EXPLAINED in Chapter 2, the standard wisdom in this field has been to take your thyroid first thing in the morning on an empty stomach and wait one hour before putting anything else in the stomach. Every experienced physician has seen a number of patients over their careers who gained weight after being started on standard thyroid treatment and report that they have food cravings. In my own practice, I can recall several patients who reported that they keep their T_4 in the bathroom because they always have to get up to go to the bathroom at 3 to 4 a.m. and, if they take their T_4 at that time, they can eat right after waking. These patients often report that they are ravenously hungry at that time. Many such patients gain weight inexorably and are told to simply eat less and exercise more.

Again, my belief is that this problem is perhaps a result of putting thyroid hormone directly on the walls of an empty stomach, thereby altering the production of such hormones as leptin and ghrelin, which are known to affect weight in humans. While it has always been taught that taking thyroid with food will reduce the percentage absorption of T_4 (thus altering thyroid balance), I have switched many such patients from taking T_4 on an empty stomach to taking it with food and most of them do not seem to notice any effect on their thyroid balance. However, I have seen a few who have become underdosed due to a reduced percentage absorption of thyroid, so one must be aware of this.

The relationship between thyroid hormone, metabolism, and weight is not as simple as often portrayed in articles on this subject. Giving supplementary thyroid hormones to encourage weight loss has been tried many times in the past, and in general, it has little or no benefit. I have seen a number of patients who have experienced gradual and substantial weight loss over a period of time on optimum treatment. However, I cannot say that I have ever made an obese person thin by simply giving thyroid hormones. Rather, I believe the weight loss is attributed to the fact that balancing thyroid levels allows the patient to reap the benefits of a dedicated program of diet and exercise.

In the past few years, I have seen some tantalizing evidence that manipulation of thyroid hormone replacement during active dieting may be of significant benefit. This is likely because T_4 is actually stored in fat tissue and is released back into the circulation during active weight loss. Additionally, when the TSH hormone is suppressed to zero by excess thyroid hormone in the circulation, it remains suppressed for long periods of time after the excess thyroid hormone is gone. Physicians will sometimes be surprised to see results showing a high T_4 and a suppressed TSH on the same dosage that the patient has used for long periods of time with normal lab results. Interpretation of such test results therefore must take into account whether there has been active weight loss or not. In such cases, the physician may assume that the patient's dose should be reduced, but a dosage reduction will actually enhance hypothyroidism at the cellular level, especially when the weight loss levels off and the patient starts to regain weight. I believe this has something to do with the commonly observed "yo-yo" phenomenon, where people lose a certain amount of weight and then regain that weight (plus a few pounds) in subsequent months. Once the weight starts returning, the flow of T_4 actually reverses, leaving muscle tissue somewhat hypothyroid. However, the TSH remains "stuck" at zero, so there is no metabolic response to the weight regaining. At this point, every pound that is regained leaves the patient's muscle tissues more hypothyroid and thus the weight regain accelerates.

I believe there is some benefit in helping patients lose weight by recognizing these changes and acting accordingly. A significant factor to consider is that TSH stimulates the activity of the T_4 to T_3 conversion enzyme at the cellular level, so pushing TSH down to zero actually reduces thyroid activity at the muscular level. If the physician is tempted to try enhancing weight loss by prescribing more thyroid, this will actually cut off the weight loss. Instead, I believe there is some benefit in reducing T_4 slightly in order to elevate the TSH and perhaps provide a bit more than the usual amount of T_3. In my practice, I now work with patients who are committed to a long-term weight loss program in which they come in for an official weekly weigh-in. If they have lost one pound or more since the previous week, I have them omit one day's T_4 dose during the following week. Again, it is important to remember that the thyroid dosage must be restored to the full level once a desired weight goal has been reached because cessation of weight loss will cut off the T_4 infusion back into the bloodstream and even a pound or two of weight gain will actually reverse the flow of T_4. These adjustments in thyroid hormone replacement have not been miraculous, but I have witnessed enough success to encourage me to continue refining this approach.

TIMING OF THYROID AND SLEEP

As described earlier, many patients have reported that their sleep improved when switching their thyroid dosage from the morning to the evening (see Chapter 2). Studies have shown that this may be due to the significant variation in TSH throughout the course of the day; this variation further undermines the TSH number as an absolute indicator of thyroid status. However, the major finding of such studies is that TSH rises sharply in the 2 to 4 hours prior to the onset of sleep. Since TSH originates in the pituitary gland of the brain and stimulates the thyroid gland to release more hormone, it certainly appears that our bodies are calling for more thyroid to be introduced into the system as we go to sleep.

When a number of my patients tried taking their mixed T_4-T_3 regimen in the evening rather than in the morning, they found that their sleep was worse and they felt overstimulated in bed at night. On their own, several of these patients determined that this must be because of the T_3, so they changed their T_3

or thyroid extract to breakfast and continued to take their T_4 at dinner. For many individuals, the improvement in sleep is gratifying, sometimes even spectacular. Nearly all patients with hypothyroidism have significant sleep disturbance with restless leg syndrome, jerking of muscles during sleep, and frequent waking, and many of my patients have found that their sleep quality improved dramatically by taking T_4 at night.

Since this regimen can be demanding and people are more likely to forget the dinner dosage, I insist that my patients lay out their T_4 pills in a 7-day pill minder. In this way, if they do miss a day, it will be obvious to them the following night, and they can take two days' worth of T_4 to keep up the overall dosing regimen. However, if the compounded capsule with T_3 or thyroid extract is missed on a given morning, I do not recommend doubling the dose the following day. A few individuals have also seen some benefit in weight management with this a.m.-p.m. regimen. The huge improvement in sleep that I have observed in many such patients raises the distinct possibility that many widespread sleep problems may actually be tied to underlying low-level hypothyroidism.

CHAPTER 15

Patients' Adjustments

IN ANOTHER chapter in this book, I proposed that the relationship between thyroid physicians and their patients should be somewhat like those between diabetes doctors and their patients. One of the huge differences I've noted between my practice and the general practice of thyroid medicine is my consideration of the distinct changes that occur seasonally. For whatever scientific reason, the fact is that patients who are in excellent balance in the summer tend to get worse in the fall and early winter, in which case an upward adjustment in dosage really helps. In the late spring, the reverse occurs, with patients again feeling fatigued because their needs have dropped and their levels are actually above the optimal point. In this situation, an interruption in T_4 and subsequent restarting at a lower dosage also has a tremendous beneficial effect.

About 15 years ago, it became clear to me that patients often came to the office in October or November complaining of feeling poorly for a month or so after feeling very well on the same thyroid regimen for months before that. Since they always complain of increased fatigue, I empirically raise their dosages even though their TSH results were not higher. Especially when the response was started with a "jumpstart" of higher dose of T_4 and then the dose reduced to perhaps 10 percent higher than before, the results were usually dramatic. After I had acquired a lot of experience with raising dosage in the fall and seeing improvement, it then became clear that the same thing in reverse happened in the late spring. Patients would typically come in to the office in May complaining of feeling very fatigued for a month or so after having had a good winter. If I stopped the T_4 for a few days and then resumed it at 10 percent or so lower, the response was just as impressive as when raising the dosage in the fall.

Interestingly, the TSH never appears to go up in the fall despite the subsequent huge improvement with an increase in dose. Correspondingly, the TSH does not go down in the spring despite the improvement on going lower on the dose. For whatever reason, patients' TSH values tend to go down in the fall and winter and go up in the spring and summer, as long as their dosage of thyroid hormone is constant. Any physician can test this out quickly in his own practice by pulling the charts of a few people who have been on the same dose of T_4 for years and comparing the TSH results from December-January-February with June-July-August. It will be very clear that all of the summer values are higher than all of the winter values. Thus, if a physician fine-tunes the T_4 dose according to which way the TSH is going, that physician will always be out of phase with the patients' needs. Once again, the TSH result is not as definitive as we have all been taught.

The almost universal occurrence of seasonal variation like

this in my practice has long fascinated me and my theory about it is as follows. If one labels results as fantastic when energy, mood, intellectual sharpness, and so on, are at 100 percent of potential, then the seasonal differences felt by the patients depend on the percentage deviation from that ideal of 100 percent. Suppose there is a 5 percent variation of your thyroid balance on a seasonal basis. If the patients are doing very poorly on 100 percent T_4 as most of them do, they might be at 60 percent of the ideal. If they fall to 55 percent on a seasonal basis, the difference from the 100 percent point is difficult to perceive. On the other hand, if someone on an excellent balanced regimen tastes 90 percent of what is possible, a seasonal drop to 85 percent represents 50 percent increase in the deviation from the ideal 100 percent.

Several of my long-time patients have been through the seasonal adjustments so frequently that they now start to do it on their own and call me only if something is not working right. My general policy is to continue the compounded capsule of T_3 or thyroid extract at one daily without exception. The T_4 increase in the fall that I routinely do is perhaps a 25-50 percent increase in $T_{4,}$ for 3 to 5 days. One might do it more gently for an older patient or someone with other medical problems. After this initial "jumpstart," I generally have them increase the dose by about 10 percent. So, if I have someone taking T_4 0.05 mg at one daily except two daily on Monday and Friday, I might well have them do three daily for 4 days and then resume dosage at one daily except for two daily on Monday, Wednesday, and Friday (MWF). I have rarely, if ever, seen any adverse effects from a "jumpstart" like this because the T_4 hormone itself is inactive, and its action in tissues is spread over a considerable period of time.

There probably are a few patients who manifest very subtle allergy problems to the T_4 pills. I have seen a few patients who report continued fatigue, achiness, and so on, with all sorts of dose manipulations and having good-looking laboratory test results. There have been a few who noted that they were dramatically better the first day that they did not take their T_4 pills. I do not believe that such a dramatic improvement results from a drop in T_4 levels but rather that such an observation implies strongly that there is something in the T_4 pills to which the patient is having some type of reaction. My first step in such patients is to simply try a different brand of T_4. If the patient gives a history of multiple sensitivities, I have the pharmacist make up T_4 in a dye-free gelatin capsule with Avicell (hypoallergenic vegetable fiber) filler.

The seasonal changes that I have just outlined are solid observations I have made over many years. For most of those years, my impression was that a colder environment required a higher amount of thyroid hormone, as if patients needed "another log on the fire." However, one of my patients recently made an interesting argument. Having successfully gone through several of these seasonal adjustments over the past few years, he raised the question of why his thyroid needs go down in May and up in September, when the average temperatures of those 2 months are roughly the same. Once again, I really don't care if the theory is correct, but the observations clearly are. One might wonder about changes in Vitamin D metabolism related more to sunlight exposure than to the ambient temperatures. Whatever the scientific basis of these observations are, it is very clear what should be done for patients complaining of symptoms at these times of the year, at least in the northern climates.

A recent exciting observation is that a number of patients on the Levothroid brand feel poorly, with fatigue, achiness, and so on, and then report that they are dramatically better even the first day by skipping the Levothroid. Such patients always seem to do much better on being switched to Levoxyl. When patients tell their physicians that they "felt better on a different brand," this is routinely dismissed, because the "different brands are the same thing." These problems with the Levothroid brand in the last year or two may well be related to reformulation, with addition of povidone to the excipient makeup. All any physician has to do to see this effect is to have the patient stop the pill for 2 days and report back if they are dramatically better. The fact that the Synthroid brand has contained povidone since its initial formulation in the 1950s raises the sad question of how many patients have been treated with Synthroid for decades and have never felt well the entire time. Physicians can get Levoxyl 50 mcg samples from the company representative and have any patient try a week or so on the dye-free pills in this particular brand.

Another area where patients can be encouraged to try another approach is in the timing of their pills. For the most part, I feel that T_3 or thyroid extract capsules should be given in the morning, since many of the patients I have had try this with the evening meal had sleep disturbances. The T_4 hormone sometimes provides remarkable benefit in sleep quality when taken with the evening meal, as discussed in Chapter 14. However, there is no one way to go here, and patients have found their comfort zone with many different regimens. I even have at least one patient who takes both T_4 and thyroid extract at bedtime and claims she has never slept better in her life. One must always consider convenience and the ability to comply so that, if a patient is frequently missing the T_4 dose with the evening meal, I have them just take both thyroid doses with breakfast.

The net result of such adjustments is to allow the physician to concentrate on the big picture and give the patient a sense of participation in his or her own care. I often tell patients that there is no one in this world who is more interested in your health than you—not your spouse, not your physician, but you.

CHAPTER 16

Compounding

COMPOUNDING T_3 or thyroid extract into time-release capsules has revolutionized my practice over the past 10 years, and this practice should become standard. (Compounding is the process by which pharmacists make up a medication specifically for an individual patient.) Giving these hormones in time-release form enhances the pharmacologic activity of the hormones, and since one can dial up any dosage in individually compounded capsules, it allows the dose to be "fine-tuned." When I switched patients from cutting Cytomel 5 mcg tablets into quarters in 1996 in favor of time-release T_3 capsules, virtually everyone was much better.

Many physicians who practice "by the book" have never written a compounded prescription, and there is some reluctance to get into completely new modes of treatment, especially if there are not some standard published studies that prove that it works. Again, let me emphasize that the dosages of T_3 or thyroid extract that I advocate are orders of magnitude lower than the doses that have already been given to tens of millions of people, so physicians should not really worry about doing this. I started doing prescriptions like this with Hopkinton Drug in the Boston area; there are other local compounding pharmacies that also do a good job. For practical purposes, compounded capsules are generally produced in units of 100, because the pharmacist uses 100 half-capsules imbedded in a small board, which he slips into his compounding table and then adds the mix, filling the half-capsules. These are the male half-capsules, and when these are filled evenly, a rack of 100 female half-capsules is then pressed on to the filled male capsules, thus creating 100 capsules.

My pharmacist has generally used a binding resin called ME4 to make the hormones time- release. In principle, the hormone sticks to this resin and then is gradually fed off as the material passes through the small bowel. Once the pharmacist has weighed out on the electronic balance 100 times the dose of T_3 or thyroid extract specified by the physician, he then adds a filler material so that the entire volume of 100 half-capsules can be filled evenly. Various fillers can be used, but the "one size fits all" material that I use is Avicell, which is hypoallergenic vegetable fiber.

The ME4 binding resin occasionally causes gastric distress in patients, perhaps about 1 percent of cases. In such an event, I try to have the capsules compounded without the ME4. While there is no time-release, at least one can pick the exact dose desired. The other alternative is to put T_3 or thyroid extract into a skin cream and have the pharmacist draw this up into 1 cc tuberculin syringes, with the concentration such that the desired dose is given in 0.1 cc of cream. I tell patients to apply this to the inner forearms. This is somewhat more costly than the capsules, so I do it only in the infrequent cases where GI distress has occurred. My general impression is that the T_3 hormone is about twice as potent when applied to the skin as it is when taken orally. Thus, to get the equivalent of a 1.0 mcg oral dose of T_3, I will prescribe T_3 cream at 5 mcg/cc, so that a 0.1 cc dose would put 0.5 mcg of T_3 on the skin. Reproduced below is a typical prescription in my practice. Since it is my standard practice to give T_3 or thyroid extract with breakfast, I usually note "cf a.m." (with food in a.m.) after one daily. The huge majority of prescriptions will work just fine with the standard ME4 binding resin and the Avicell filler material, which I abbreviate "M/Av." There may well be useful alternative binders and fillers to use in a given case, so the physician is encouraged to discuss this with his local compounding pharmacist.

As I have outlined in the rest of this book, getting the dosages of T_4 and T_3 right for a given individual is the key to success in this area. When a physician gains significant experience in doing this, it makes she or he realize how completely off the mark the various trials with rigid overdoses of T_3 were. Many other physicians have been prescribing T_3 in time-release capsules in the past few years, and when such a patient comes to me later, the mistake that has always been made is giving too much T_3. As discussed in Chapter 5, the official therapeutic trials of adding T_3 to T_4 used dosages of T_3 that represent a 10-fold to 20-fold overdose. Not surprisingly, they concluded that T_3 made people worse rather than better. A META analysis (*JCEM* 91:2592, 2006) has been published recently on the T_3 trials that I have referred to in this book, and not surprisingly, they concluded that there was no role for T_3 in the treatment of hypothyroidism. A META-analysis amounts to a statistical averaging of different studies on the same subject and can be helpful when the individual studies do not agree. To actually do a META-analysis of six studies that all say the same thing represents a new high (or low) in redundant academic publishing. This is a new category of paper, a "quadruple-blind" study, since the editor who accepted this paper had to be blind as well.

Considering that an individual pharmacist is making one bottle of capsules for one patient, one wonders about the possibility of making a mistake. When a standard drug is run off the production lines at a major pharmaceutical manufacturer, there is a great deal of quality control and lot numbers to prevent major errors. Most of my prescriptions for the last 10 years or so have been done at Hopkinton Drug in Hopkinton, Massachusetts, but there are several other compounding pharmacies that also appear to do a good job.

Many practicing physicians have never used compounding so there is a bit of "getting over the hump" to doing so. What follows is a typical prescription of what I would prescribe for a patient who has good thyroid test numbers while taking 50 mcg daily of T_4.

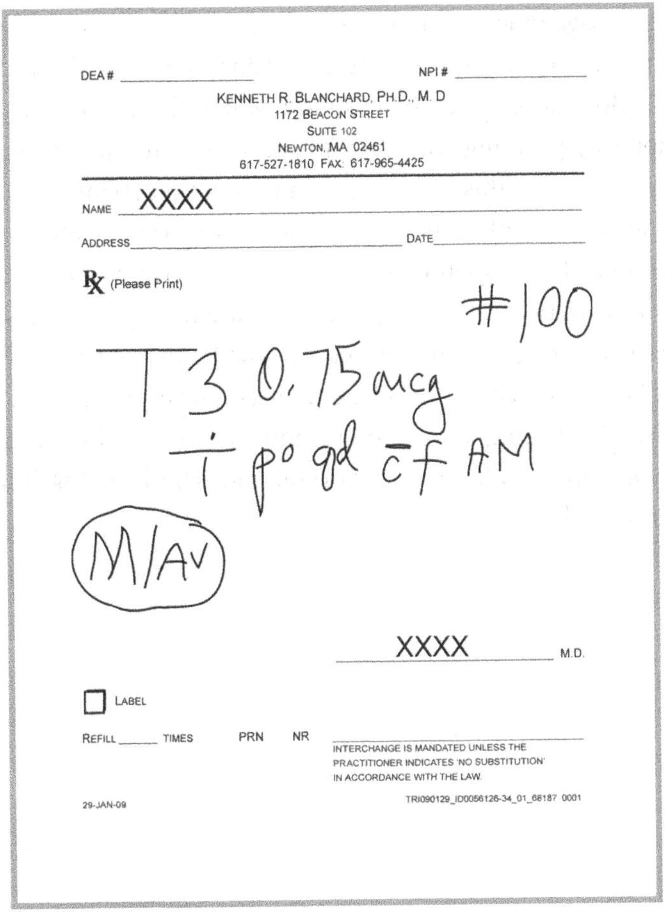

DEA # ______________ NPI # ______________

KENNETH R. BLANCHARD, PH.D., M. D
1172 BEACON STREET
SUITE 102
NEWTON, MA 02461
617-527-1810 FAX: 617-965-4425

NAME XXXX

ADDRESS ______________ DATE ______________

℞ (Please Print)

#100

T3 0.75 mcg
i po qd c̄ AM

M/AV

XXXX M.D.

☐ LABEL

REFILL ____ TIMES PRN NR

INTERCHANGE IS MANDATED UNLESS THE PRACTITIONER INDICATES 'NO SUBSTITUTION' IN ACCORDANCE WITH THE LAW.

29-JAN-09

TRI090129_ID0056126-34_01_68187 0001

To get the 98.5:1.5 T_4:T_3 ratio that is a reasonable starting point, this patient would get a dose of T_3 0.75 mcg in time-release form. Writing a prescription like this should not cause much consternation for the prescribing physician, since the dosages that I recommend are orders of magnitude lower than the amounts of T_3 that have already been given historically. Recall that the recent spate of "T_3 does not work" papers used daily dosage ranges of 6 to 25 mcg. The results are not much different whether one gives a 5-fold overdose or a 10-fold overdose of T_3. Both doses give a bad result. I would like to conclude this chapter by pleading with thyroid specialists, and physicians in general, to give this a try. When a desperate patient comes to you feeling terrible although they are taking 100 percent T_4 and have good-looking laboratory test results, please do not recite to them the outworn teachings that "you are on thyroid and your TSH is normal, so your symptoms can't be thyroid-related" or that "nobody needs T_3 because T_4 gets converted to T_3 in the body." Try writing a few prescriptions like this and then make up your mind as far as who is right and who is wrong in this ongoing debate.

CHAPTER 17

Transdermal Thyroid

IT WAS clear soon after starting to use compounded time-release capsules of T_3 that there are a few people (probably less than 1 percent) who have gastric upset on these capsules. Rarely, the GI distress is related to the use of natural thyroid extract; most often it is due to the ME4 binding resin that makes the hormone time-release. Because of this problem, I started having my compounding pharmacist make T_3 into a skin cream which he draws up into 1 cc tuberculin syringes, allowing easy measurement of 0.1 cc of cream. I generally have patients apply this to the inner forearms. There is no doubt that this method of giving T_3 works quite well, but the prescriptions are somewhat more expensive than the time-release capsules.

Since I have long been suspicious that direct contact of thyroid hormone with the walls of the stomach might contribute to weight gain, I thought that patients might possibly do better weight-wise by using transdermal thyroid, thus eliminating any thyroid-gastric wall contact. However, as often seems to be the case with any gimmicks for weight loss, this has unfortunately not held up over time. Going further in this area, I even tried creams with both T_4 and T_3 in the mix, but this treatment failed miserably. There were only a few such patients, and they typically came back feeling very poorly, with a low T_4 and a high TSH. At first I questioned my compounding pharmacist as to whether he had forgotten to put the T_4 into the cream, but I was always assured otherwise. Then I consulted a compounding guru in Houston, who reported to me that giving T_4 in a skin cream has been tried many times and it never seems to work. After going through all of this, a simple review of the basic thyroid physiology gives the obvious answer. The deiodinase enzyme in the body that clips iodines off the molecular structure of the T_4 hormone exists in three different forms, labeled I, II and III. The type III deiodinase enzyme is very prominent in human skin, and this particular enzyme specifically converts T_4 into reverse T_3, which is inactive.

One advantage of using T_3 in a skin cream is that it is very easy to try small increments or decrements in the dose to assess response. In other words, if a patient is doing poorly and I want to see the result of increasing the proportion of T_3, I often have patients use 0.15 cc of T_3 per day as a trial. Since the effect of an increase in T_3 becomes evident very early, it usually does not take more than a few days or a week at most to decide if this adjustment is beneficial or not. Correspondingly, if my guess is that the T_3 level is too high, I often have people drop it back to 0.05 cc daily. Doing these relatively large percentage changes very quickly determines whether the direction in which the T_3 is going is the right one or not.

I have also tried having natural thyroid extract put in the skin cream. The practical problem with this approach is the rather unpleasant smell of thyroid extract. It is not overwhelming, so if there were a huge advantage in using thyroid extract, it is still doable. However, I have not seen any major advantage in using thyroid extract in a cream form as opposed to T_3, so there are only a few patients in my practice on this preparation. There is also the theoretical disadvantage of having the type III deiodinase enzyme in skin converting the T_4 in the extract into reverse T_3, which may have an adverse effect on thyroid balance.

CHAPTER 18

How to Do It

THIS CHAPTER is meant to be a practical guide to physicians and their empowered patients for treating hypothyroidism in an optimal way.

Frequently, physicians see patients with a long history highly suggestive of hypothyroidism, perhaps with some strong physical findings of hypothyroidism, but "normal tests." My belief is that all such patients should be given a therapeutic trial on 25 mcg of T_4, which I believe is much safer and more natural than giving antidepressants, sleeping pills, or stimulant drugs. My preference is to give Levoxyl 0.05 mg at one-half tablet daily for a two to three week trial. When they have a major degree of sleep disturbance (as they often do), I have them take the dose with the evening meal for a few days to assess the effect on sleep. There usually is a distinct sleep benefit, often on the very first night of treatment. Since taking it at this time of day is difficult for compliance over the long term, I have them switch it back to breakfast in a few days and keep it there, as long as the sleep benefit is not lost. I generally have the patients report back on the results of the trial by 2 to 3 weeks. What happens quite often is that the benefit in regard to energy tops out at one week or so, and they report that the effect is slipping. This is the classic "up and down" phenomenon. The key question at this point is whether they need more $T_{4,}$ or some T_3 should be added. Since the ultimate goal in treatment is to establish the correct T_4:T_3 ratio, I believe the next step is to increase the T_4, perhaps to 25 mcg daily except 50 mcg MWF. If the patient then reports feeling no better or even worse, my belief is that this indicates a need for the T_3 hormone. In essence, what we are doing is increasing the T_4:T_3 ratio with the higher dose of T_4 and thus a worsening clinical state strongly implies the need for the T_3 hormone.

A minority of patients will continue to feel very well on 100 percent T_4, and in that case, I will leave them on that regimen. My observation is that young people who exercise a great deal may indeed be well treated with 100 percent T_4, presumably because exercise enhances T_4 to T_3 conversion in tissues, resulting in a favorable T_4:T_3 balance at the cellular level.

For those individuals who report that they are worse on the higher dose of the T_4, I have them drop the T_4 back to 25 mcg daily and add at T_3 0.3 to 0.4 mcg or thyroid extract at 2 to 2.5 mg daily. These patients can show amazing results very quickly with the addition of T_3, especially if "brain fog" is a major problem. As mentioned elsewhere, the institution of time-release T_3 causes the body to "use T_4 faster" and so these patients will very frequently show the "up and down" effect again after a few weeks. This should be addressed by an increase in the T_4 dose, for example, 25 mcg daily except for 50 mcg Monday and Friday.

Most patients treated this way will feel extremely well for a period of time after the establishment of this dosage regimen. Especially if treatment is being initiated in the fall and winter when there is increasing need, they will often call back and report that they have become very fatigued again. The answer in almost every such case is to give more T_4. What I do generally is to give them a "jumpstart" of 50 mcg daily for three or 4 days, then reduce it to 25 mcg daily except 50 mcg MWF. The reason I do this is there is a very large T_4 pool in the body and the half-life of T_4 is about a week, so minor changes in T_4 dose will not be observed in a week or two. With the "jumpstart," they will often feel much better by 2 weeks, which therefore proves that the adjustment was the correct one.

A very common clinical presentation in my practice is a patient who was diagnosed a few years before by the clinical picture and elevated TSH and was started on 100 percent T_4 and has experienced the "up and down" phenomenon. They remember improving dramatically for perhaps 2 to 3 months on 100 percent T_4 and keep coming back after that complaining of a return of hypothyroid symptoms. The usual physician response is that "you are on thyroid and your TSH is normal, so your complaints cannot be related to thyroid." Indeed, the "up and down" phenomenon is what dictates the need for T_3. If a patient comes to me on a dose of T_4 where the TSH is fairly optimal, for example, at 1.5, I keep them on the same dose of T_4 and add T_3 or thyroid extract in such proportions as to give a 98.5:1.5 ratio. If the patient for instance is taking 50 mcg T_4, this means that they need a T_3 capsule of about 0.75 mcg or 5 mg of thyroid extract. These are the easiest patients that I ever see, and the results are almost universally and dramatically beneficial. I have pleaded in vain with several academic leaders to assign a fellow or resident to observe what I do and see what happens to patients like this, but I have always been dismissed because there are "no studies." Interested physicians with open minds are encouraged to try the techniques that I have outlined in this chapter. All of us worry about being sued if something goes wrong, but just consider that the dosages of T_3 and thyroid extract that I advocate are orders of magnitude lower than what has already been taken by tens of millions of people. Older patients often come in having been on two grains of thyroid extract for 30 years. This amount of thyroid extract supplies about 18 mcg of T_3, which is about 15 times the average dose that I use in my practice. Many physicians have also tried Cytomel 5 or 10 mcg daily and observed the responses that I have documented elsewhere in this book: initial positive response and then complete failure. For the details of writing these prescriptions, individual physicians should consult with local compounding pharmacists, but it is very easy to become accustomed to this approach, and for those physicians willing to open their minds, the results will be amazing.

I have found it very helpful to use a linear graph of mcg of T_3 versus mg of thyroid extract to calculate the dosages of the capsules. Since there is about 2.2 mcg of T_3 in 15 mg of thyroid extract, that point along with the zero point establishes the linear relationship. One can figure out the amount of T_3 that one wants to give with a given dose of T_4 and find that on the ordinate and then simply go across to the line and then downward to find the amount of extract that is equivalent to it.

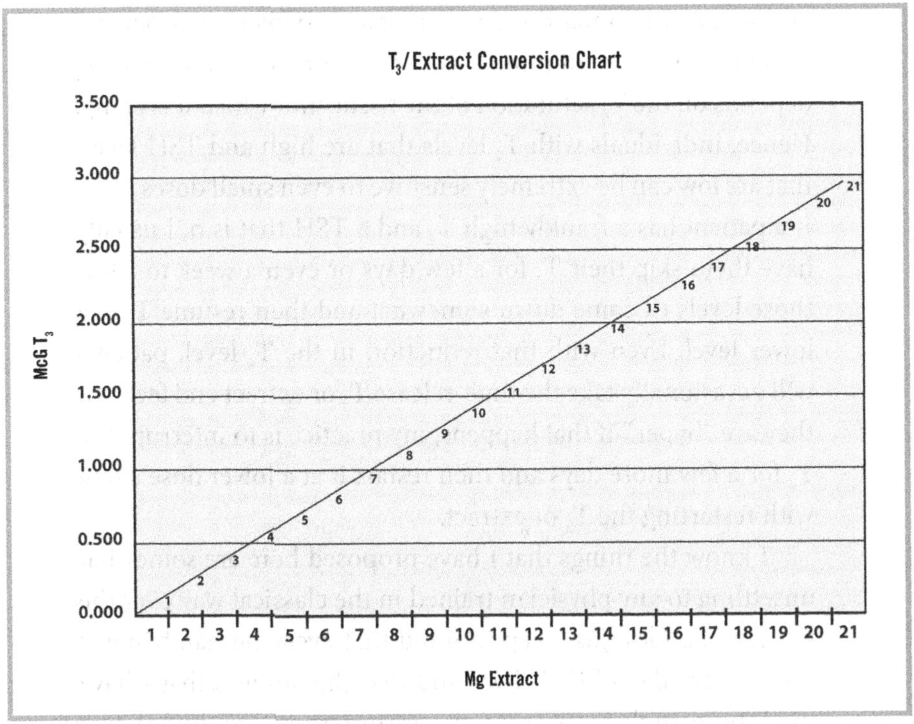

For instance, if a patient has good laboratory numbers on 50 mcg of T_4, then I would generally start them on 0.75 mcg of T_3, which according to the graph means 5 mg of thyroid extract. In general, I determine the T_4 dose predominantly by the laboratory test results; then the trick to getting people feeling better is the decision of how much T_3 to put with that amount of T_4. My general starting point is 98.5 percent T_4:1.5 percent T_3, but I might well shave those portions one way or the other depending on other factors. I believe that one has to respect the patient's report that "I am very sensitive to medications" and go low on the initial dosage, perhaps 99 percent T_4:1 percent T_3. One must keep in mind that the effect of a given dose of T_3 depends on the T_4 saturation of the tissue into which it is going. Hence, individuals with T_4 levels that are high and TSH levels that are low can be extremely sensitive to even small doses of T_3. If a patient has a frankly high T_4 and a TSH that is 0, I usually have them skip their T_4 for a few days or even a week to allow those levels to come down somewhat and then resume T_4 at a lower level. Even with that reduction in the T_4 level, patients will occasionally take the time-release T_3 or extract and feel that they are "hyper." If that happens, my practice is to interrupt the T_4 for a few more days and then restart it at a lower dose along with restarting the T_3 or extract.

I know the things that I have proposed here are somewhat unsettling to any physician trained in the classical way over the last few decades. Just keep in mind that every human being is on T_3 every day of their lives and that the dosages that I have used successfully for over 15 years are orders of magnitude lower than dosages that have already been taken by tens of millions of people.

CHAPTER 19

Future Trials

THERE ARE a number of potential studies that could be done in the future by researchers with open minds who are dedicated to doing better for our patients. In my experience, the nature of a thyroid replacement and the timing of that replacement has been extremely important in sleep quality for my patients. As outlined elsewhere in this book, the optimum regimen for many patients is to take T_4 pills with the evening meal and T_3 or thyroid extract with breakfast. It would be of interest to repeat the prior experiments drawing hourly TSH on volunteers in the evening and early sleep hours. Since TSH comes from the brain and stimulates the thyroid gland to release more thyroid hormone, the rise in TSH prior to the onset of sleep suggests that our natural biorhythms call for more thyroid to be introduced into the system at that time. Besides TSH, the other hormones of interest would be melatonin and growth hormone. The idea would be to compare what happens to these hormones when a patient takes T_4 with the evening meal versus taking it in the morning. I suspect that taking T_4 in the hours approaching sleep increases the release of melatonin and growth hormone and thus enhances the benefit of this type of treatment.

It is of interest that as late as the 1960s, hypothyroidism was felt to be a major risk factor for breast cancer. The idea at the time was that, in studies of lifetime drug histories, women presenting with breast cancer were several times more likely to be on thyroid hormone than women with other diagnoses. Of course, in those days, a few patients were diagnosed by the cumbersome and expensive Basal Metabolic Rate Test, but many were just empirically treated with thyroid on the basis of the judgment of the physician. When the TSH test came into vogue in the 1970s and all physicians were admonished that this was the "modern" and "scientific" way of diagnosing hypothyroidism, a new era in thyroid research was born. We were taught that the TSH is the absolute measure of thyroid function, and many things were then investigated measuring TSH levels in patients with specific diagnoses and assuming that if the average TSH of a given group of patients was the same as in the general population, then the problem of that group could not be related to thyroid. It turns out that if one measures TSH levels in large numbers of women presenting with breast cancer, the TSH is in fact not significantly different from that in the general population. For that reason, hypothyroidism has not been mentioned in the same discussion with breast cancer for over 30 years. Though far from a scientific statistical fact, my overall observation over the past 30 years has been that I have seen far less breast cancer than would have been expected. For that reason, I personally believe that the proper treatment of hypothyroidism probably does help to prevent the development of breast cancer. If there is any truth to this, the reason for that may be that the proper thyroid treatment enhances the release of melatonin at the time of falling asleep. Melatonin deficiency is now on the radar as a potential factor in the development of breast cancer. The possible role of melatonin in breast cancer was raised by the higher incidence of this disease in nurses who did more night shifts, which does disrupt normal melatonin production.

Another interesting area for experimentation would be to note what happens to TSH early in the course of empirical treatment of patients with clinical hypothyroidism but normal TSH. Standard wisdom would say that the normal TSH would be further suppressed possibly into the "toxic" range by oral thyroid, yet if the thyroid is given in the proper dosage, in most cases the TSH actually rises with thyroid supplementation. This is something that I have observed many times in my practice. Of course, if someone starts a patient with normal TSH on 100 mcg of T_4 daily, as has been done in some empirical studies in the past, they will indeed suppress their TSH below normal because of the overdose. However, if such patients are given a more-physiologic 25-mcg dose, I predict that the TSH will actually go up in many. Following the type of adjustments detailed in Chapter 15, the patient may well be taking both T_4 and thyroid extract, and yet have a TSH higher than they had when they took no thyroid. This is a phenomenon which is impossible to explain by standard teachings in the field. I believe that this phenomenon is caused by the activity of the Type-I deiodinase enzyme in the pituitary gland, which is causing T_4 to T_3 conversion within the gland itself. It is well known that the activity of this enzyme is enhanced in the presence of hypothyroidism. Indeed, I believe that it is a compensatory measure instituted by the body to try to overcome the effects of inadequate T_4 levels.

In other words, as T_4 production falls in the failing gland and T_4 levels start to decline, reasonably normal T_3 levels in the tissues are maintained by accelerating the T_4 to T_3 conversion. For example, one might have tissue T_4 levels that are 30 percent below optimum, but the T_3 levels in the tissues might be just 5 percent low. This explains the phenomenon that all experienced physicians have seen, having the TSH come back very high at 50 to 100 mIU/L and then being amazed that the patient is still standing up. This is because TSH itself is a regulator of the Type-I deiodinase enzyme and is extremely rapidly converting T_4 to T_3 in that situation. Thus, the symptoms of hypothyroidism are being ameliorated considerably. When such patients are treated with the standard T_4, they will often have remarkable benefits for a month or two and then, when the TSH is suppressed to lower levels, for example, to 1.0, the symptoms of hypothyroidism come back again. I believe that this is because of the suppression of TSH on treatment, which is turning down the T_4 to T_3 conversion peripherally in tissues. This is the situation in which many new patients come to me for treatment. If basic T_4 and TSH values look good, I add T_3 or thyroid extract so as to give about a 98.5:1.5 T_4:T_3 ratio and continue the same dose of T_4 as before. Since there is some T_4 in thyroid extract, the T_4 dose is actually *increased* with the addition of T_3. I do not recall a single patient who ever developed symptoms of overdose following this protocol. It is as if the improved metabolism causes the body to use T_4 faster.

Another possibly fruitful area for research is empirical treatment of hypothyroidism in patients with major sleep disorders, but normal thyroid tests. This includes the "restless leg syndrome (RLS)," for which an expensive patented drug has recently been introduced. This drug may well work for many individuals, but it makes more sense to actually correct the underlying thyroid problem that is in fact the cause of RLS. We have all seen newsmagazine cover stories indicating the vast extent of sleep disorders in our society. This would be impossible for most conventional thinkers to swallow, but I would propose giving any sleep disorder patient 25 mcg of T_4 with the evening meal to see if it works. The academicians will say that this is overdiagnosing hypothyroidism and seeing hypothyroidism everywhere, but there is nothing to be lost by such a simple therapeutic trial of even a week or two. In my experience, most such patients noticed a distinct improvement in sleep quality the very first night when they take T_4 with the evening meal. The alternative has been a series of expensive drugs that often cause many problems, such as dependence and cognitive impairment. In a sense, resolution of a sleep disorder in this way would be a "functional" way of diagnosing hypothyroidism. I have no idea what the response rate would be, but I guarantee that it would be higher than just a few percent. This type of treatment would be orders of magnitude less expensive and much safer than the sleep drugs now in use.

Given the high prevalence of premenstrual syndrome and its terrible toll on both women and their families, the relationship of thyroid to PMS should be explored further. As outlined in Chapter 8, I have had enormous success in moderately increasing T_4 dosage and stopping T_3 during a week or so of PMS. Even in women who do not appear to be clinically hypothyroid enough to commit them to taking thyroid hormone, it would be very simple to give a group of volunteers with severe PMS 25 mcg of T_4 for perhaps 10 days each month leading up to the onset of menstrual flow. I have not specifically had experience in doing this since patients in my practice are there for the treatment of hypothyroidism, but I think it is extremely likely that this simple treatment would work beautifully. If it does, it probably would identify a group of women who eventually should be on permanent thyroid treatment for optimal health. As discussed in Chapter 8, the formal academic studies on the relationship between thyroid function and PMS published in the early 1990s both had the fatal flaw of using 100 mcg of T_4 as empirical treatment. Some of the subjects in those studies probably remember feeling notably better for a week or two as the thyroid levels normalized, but the benefit quickly faded as they went right through the "sweet spot" and became overdosed. This points out again that thyroid supplementation is fundamentally an attempt to restore normal body physiology by giving the optimum dose with no benefit observed by going above the optimum point; in fact, most often the same symptoms reappear above the optimum dose as existed before treatment. When such a patient asks why she had a week or two of feeling great before she started to feel poorly, this is dismissed as a "placebo response." Academicians like to design studies with numerous rigid criteria, but the difference in doses needed by individuals and whether they also need some T_3 or not make these studies unrealistic. Any future study in this area has to respect individually designed thyroid replacement requirements rather than another "designed to fail" trial of "thyroid versus placebo."

CHAPTER 20

The T_4:T_3 Ratio

My firm belief at this point in my career is that the T_4:T_3 ratio in the body tissues determines the result that a patient experiences with regard to thyroid treatment. The various factors which determine this are the amounts of T_4 and T_3 being secreted from the thyroid gland and the subsequent metabolism of T_4 and T_3 within body tissues. For a person taking thyroid hormone, there are the relative absorptions of the T_4 and T_3 hormones to consider as well as subsequent metabolic change occurring in the liver before these hormones reach the bloodstream. Studies have shown that the T_3 hormone is better absorbed than T_4. When one considers all the variables involved here, it becomes clear that simple formulas for giving thyroid hormone cannot exist. Hence, the need for the functional approach to this problem, as I have indicated elsewhere.

The spectrum of oral thyroid replacement in humans runs from the standard 100 percent T_4 through the 80 percent: 20 percent ratio seen in natural thyroid extract. The standard academic wisdom states that T_3 is an unnecessary treatment. However, this ignores the fact that T_3 which is secreted into the bloodstream by the thyroid gland is a different pool of T_3 in the body from that which is generated from T_4 within body tissues. My belief is that the optimum T_4:T_3 percentage in humans is represented by the accompanying graph.

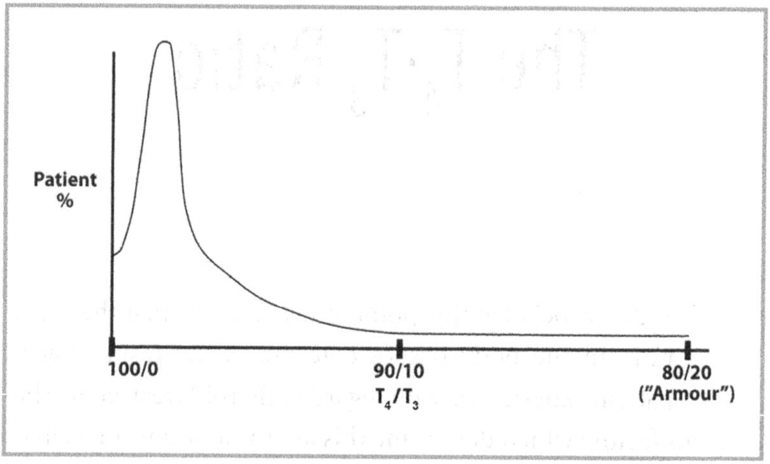

With the overwhelming number of patients optimal in the 98.5 percent to 99 percent T_4:1 percent to 1.5 percent T_3, an important thing to keep in mind in approaching this question is that TSH is a stimulator of the peripheral Type-I deiodinase enzyme in tissues, which is one of the main reasons why patients who have had thyroid ablation (by surgery or radioactive iodine) feel so poorly. They are usually overloaded with T_4, and the low TSH is inhibiting T_3 generation within tissues, hence they have a very high T_4:T_3 ratio at tissue level.

In giving the patients T_4-T_3 mixtures, one often sees initial excellent response and then a worsening in the patient's condition (the "up and down" phenomenon). In the patients who come to my practice who have taken T_3 in the past, the almost universal mistake made in their treatment was to give too much T_3. Since T_3 is said to be the direct-acting hormone, the natural instinct of the physician when told by the patient that fatigue is increasing is to increase the amount of T_3. However, my experience is that the way to adjust over time is a gradual *increase* of the T_4:T_3 ratio, which means raising T_4 (if the TSH is not too low already) or reducing T_3.

If the patient experiences a period of time with a wonderful result, one can safely assume that they are at an optimal T_4:T_3 ratio. In such a circumstance, raising T_3 rarely will cause an improvement in energy and other responses but rather will make the patient feel worse. Because the ultimate desirable situation is the ideal T_4:T_3 ratio, raising the T_3 in this circumstance "creates a relative deficit of T_4."

One can now understand why the numerous studies concluding "T_3 makes people worse rather than better" arrived at their result, since the doses given typically resulted in T_4:T_3 ratios of 70:30, 60:40, and so on.

The nature of a patient's hypothyroidism is extremely important in determining the ideal T_4:T_3 ratio. Patients fall on a spectrum from a very slight degree of hypothyroidism in an intact thyroid gland to a total loss of endogenous secretion due to thyroid ablation. Since patients with thyroid ablation have lost all their secreted T_3, they may well need a significantly higher percentage of oral T_3 in their regimen for optimal physiologic effect. Many patients come to me who have been tried on various forms of T_3 and have records including many T_3 and free T_3 lab tests. My belief is that these tests are totally useless because of considerable variation in blood levels depending on when the last T_3 dose was taken. Here again, my belief is that the optimum T_3 dose can only be ascertained by the functional approach. What I do is to take the typical ablation patient on 100 percent T_4 and give them about 98 percent T_4:2 percent T_3 initial treatment and then gradually work the T_3 percentage higher over a period of time as long as the patient keeps improving. One should always keep in mind that the institution of time-release T_3 improves the patient's metabolism such that they appear to use their T_4 faster. This is the reason why the standard practice of reducing T_4 by 4 mcg for every 1 mcg of T_3 given is totally wrong.

Physicians will very often have patients come in to see them on this type of treatment who have TSH results well below normal; technically, they have been overdosed. They usually feel only fatigued rather than the classic "hyper" symptoms such as palpitation and shakiness. When patients have been overdosed in the past, pushing the TSH down to zero, the TSH almost always seems to "get stuck." One can reduce the dosages of T_4 and T_3 considerably, even enough to increase hypothyroid symptoms, and the TSH will continue to be low. A physician evaluating a patient under those circumstances would probably feel there is still overdose and lower the dosage more. Hence, my belief is that there should be mild reductions of both T_4 and T_3 to allow time for the TSH to become "unstuck," as long as there are no symptoms suggesting overdose.

When one considers the fact that most patients are ideally treated with T_3 in the 0.5 to 1.5 mcg daily dose range, one realizes how far off the mark are the academic studies that are negative on T_3, with their dosages of 6 to 25 mcg daily. Anyone who gains some experience in doing T_3 this way will greatly appreciate how tiny percentage changes in T_3 dose can cause dramatic differences in symptoms. Taking this factor into account also points out how difficult it would be to do standard academic double-blind placebo-controlled studies with fixed doses of T_3. Such studies would be like doing trials on diabetics with placebos versus fixed doses of insulin. One does not have to be an academic expert to recognize that fixed dosages in situations like this cannot result in a good, definitive study result.

The other end of the T_3-T_4 spectrum are the patients with very mild degrees of hypothyroidism. These are often patients who show positive TPO antibodies, thus the designation of Hashimoto's disease, an autoimmune disorder of the thyroid gland. Those patients who have a good clinical response to just 25 mcg or so of T_4 very often do not need T_3, because their intact gland is still producing adequate amounts of T_3. Here again, the only way to know for sure is to do it the functional way, that is, optimized treatment with $T_{4,}$ and if the response is less than great, try a small dose of T_3. If someone is on a dose of T_3 and there is real question whether the T_3 is doing any good, what I would do is have them stop the T_3 when they have a few capsules left and see if symptoms like brain fog, sleep disturbance, and fatigue increase quickly. If they do, resumption of the remaining T_3 capsules will give a rapid positive response, the functional approach again. Another corollary of this observation on patients with minimal hypothyroidism is that they clearly have a much better chance of being well replaced with 100 percent T_4.

For those physicians who see thyroid ablation patients who are on a dose of $T_{4,}$ indicating that that they are fully replaced, although they feel terrible, I would plead with you to just try writing a compound capsule in the appropriate dose range to see what happens. If a patient, for instance, looks to be adequately replaced with 150 mcg of T_4, write a compounded capsule of thyroid extract at 15 mg and add it to the T_4. Do this on a couple of patients and I promise that you will feel regrets over the standard practice of giving 100 percent T_4.

CHAPTER 21

Conclusion

In summary, I would state that there has never been a situation in the history of medicine where fundamentally wrong teachings have held sway for so many years and hurt the quality of life of so many patients. The teachings in this field that a "normal TSH rules out hypothyroidism" and "nobody needs T_3 because T_4 turns into T_3," continue to be taught in medical schools. As my own career has been winding down, I have long sought a young endocrinologist to join me and gradually take over my practice, but few have even been willing to come in and talk to me. One who did talk to me, said "Dr. Blanchard, everything you do is wrong, so if I joined you I would be a professional outcast and get sued." Well, I have never been sued and my practice is incredibly successful and draws many of the former patients of the academic leaders whom they believed have all the answers. My hope at this time is that conscientious physicians who are capable of getting their minds "outside the box" will at least consider the ideas that I have espoused in this book. Try some of the simple things that I have indicated at first to convince yourself that I really know what I am talking about. For people taking T_4 in the morning and who have serious sleep problems, just try having them take the T_4 with the evening meal. If you do, probably three of five will be distinctly better and one or two will consider it a miracle. Just note how often you make a classic diagnosis, start someone on T_4, and they then proceed to exhibit the "up and down" phenomenon over the next few months. If you are willing to open your minds and make observations like this, you will conclude that I know what I am talking about and perhaps will venture into prescribing time-release T_3 and/or thyroid extract. Any physician who embraces the ideas in this book will have a very rewarding practice. You will have extremely grateful patients and have the honor of people learning about your practice by word of mouth and coming to see you from great distances. I truly do hope that the ideas of this book will catch on so my current patients will not feel that my impending retirement means the end of their good results and their healthier and more satisfying life.

About the Author

KENNETH R. BLANCHARD, M.D., PH.D. is an endocrinologist certified by The American Board of Internal Medicine and The American Board of Endocrinology and Metabolism. His undergraduate degree was at MIT and he received a Ph.D. in chemistry from Princeton University. He taught chemistry at Vassar College for three years before going on to Cornell University Medical College. He trained for 2 years at New York–Memorial Hospitals in New York City and then completed a fellowship in endocrinology at the Boston VA Hospital. Dr. Blanchard also practiced general internal medicine until 2000 and now concentrates only on thyroid disease and menopausal hormone replacement therapy. He has been in private practice in Newton, Massachusetts, from 1976 to the present time. He has done numerous magazine, radio, and TV interviews in recent years. He is the father of two sons and his wife, Rita, is also a physician. They continue to live in Newton.